Advanced praise for Taekwondo – A Path to Excellence...

"I was deeply impressed by your eloquence in bringing to life the tenets and rich history of Taekwondo. Your work is utterly outstanding and informative and beautifully captures the art of Taekwondo as a way of life that encompasses the mind, body, and spirit seeking total perfection.

"I would like to applaud you for your dedication to this work of passing on the culture, history, and art that is Taekwondo. I highly recommend your book to not only Taekwondo practitioners but to all serious students of the martial arts.

"It has been a deep pleasure to read your book."

> —Grandmaster Hee Il Cho, AIMMA President and Founder

"Thank you for sending me your manuscript on *Taekwondo—A Path to Excellence.* I have read your previous books and truly feel that they are some of the best material presented on Taekwondo that I have ever read in my 39 years of studying and practicing martial arts.

"In today's martial arts world, you are a voice that must be heard. As a fellow Taekwondo practitioner, I sincerely thank you for providing the martial arts community with such an outstanding book that encompasses every aspect of the traditional art of Taekwondo.

"I am mandating that all my black belt students read and give a thesis on your book!"

> —Master Philip Ameris, 7th dan black belt, Technical Director, Action International Martial Arts Association

"Master Cook has done it again! Over the years I have read dozens of books on Taekwondo, but this one is my favorite. It inspires, informs, motivates, and entertains from beginning to end. This book presents an in-depth analysis of the many facets and manifestations of Taekwondo, providing new insight and appreciation for the art for beginner students and seasoned instructors alike. A truly enjoyable and educational read."

> —Grandmaster John Pellegrini, 9th dan, President and Founder of the Independent Taekwondo Association and International Combat Hapkido Federation

"Doing and telling are not the same, but Doug Cook's newest book reveals a martial arts teacher as skilled in the use of the pen as he is with the arts of the dojang. *Taekwondo—A Path to Excellence* is a well-conceived and skillfully written invitation to explore the oft-neglected traditional and philosophical aspects of taekwondo. As such, it is a refreshing change of pace. Readers will benefit from the author's extensive experience in training and his profound insight regarding its purpose. The book, like the art itself, is conceived by Mr. Cook as a journey where disciplined practice leads to spiritual enrichment. Readers who pick up this nicely written volume will find that they have taken yet another step toward this worthwhile goal."

—John Donohue, Ph.D., best-selling author of martial arts books and fiction

"*Taekwondo—A Path to Excellence* puts the Do back in Taekwondo. As the author skillfully argues by weaving together history, philosophy, and modern practice, Taekwondo is not simply a set of skills evidenced by a set of colored belts. It is a noble Do, a way of life, grounded in the most profound values."

—Mark K. Setton, Associate Professor, Chairman of Martial Arts Studies, University of Bridgeport, CT

"Written by one of its leading practitioners, *Taekwondo—A Path to Excellence* is a fascinating look into the system's history, practice, and philosophy."

—Michael Rosenbaum, Chief Instructor, Snow Leopard Boxing Fist, best-selling author of martial arts books

"In his third book, Doug Cook has once again made an excellent contribution to his art, penning a tome that should prove relevant, interesting, and important for taekwondo practitioners everywhere. In the 2008 Olympic Games many of us watched with revulsion as competitor Angel Matos pushed a judge, kicked the referee in the face, and spit on the floor before stalking out after he was disqualified in his bronze-medal match. While both he and his coach Leudis Gonzalez were subsequently banned for life, the incident clearly points out a distressing lack in these individuals' training. It is refreshing to find a book with emphasis on the original philosophical and combative components of the art, rather than solely on the sporting aspects as is all too common in many dojang these days. As the title implies, Master Cook truly has outlined a path to excellence, one where the practice of Taekwondo can lead to physical and spiritual enrichment. It is a great read!"

—Lawrence A. Kane, Sensei, Security Professional, best-selling author of martial arts books

Taekwondo

a path to excellence

Taekwondo
a path to excellence

DOUG COOK

YMAA Publication Center
Wolfeboro, N.H., USA

YMAA Publication Center
Main Office: PO Box 480
Wolfeboro, NH 03894
1-800-669-8892 • www.ymaa.com • info@ymaa.com

ISBN: 9781594391286 (print) • ISBN: 9781594392054 (ebook)

Cover design by Axie Breen
Edited by Barbara Langley
Photographs by the author unless otherwise noted.

YMAA Publication Center strives to conform this book's editorial to the Chicago Manual of Style 15th edition with the following exceptions. Foreign words either common or uncommon have been italicized at their first appearance, with subsequent appearances generally non-italic. The words 'do' and 'The Way' have retained italics throughout. The word 'Ki' is capitalized throughout. Other uses of italics may be for author's emphasis.

Publisher's Cataloging in Publication
Cook, Doug.

    Taekwondo : a path to excellence / Doug Cook. --Wolfeboro,
N.H. : YMAA Publication Center, c2009.

      p. ; cm.
      ISBN: ISBN-13: 978-1-59439-128-6 ; ISBN-10:
1-59439-128-9
      "Achieving physical and spiritual enrichment through
disciplined practice."--Cover.
      Includes bibliographical references and index.

      1. Tae kwon do--Philosophy. 2. Tae kwon do--Moral and
ethical aspects. 3. Martial arts--Moral and ethical aspects.
4. Martial artists--Conduct of life. I. Title. II. Title: Tae kwon do.

GV1114.9 .C668 2009   2009936408
796.815/3--dc22   0910

POD 0417

Disclaimer. The author and publisher of this material are NOT RESPONSIBLE in any manner whatsoever for any injury which may occur through reading or following the instructions in this manual. The activities, physical or otherwise, described in this material may be too strenuous or dangerous for some people and the reader(s) should consult a physician before engaging in them.

    The author wishes to assure the reader that the use of personal pronouns "he" or "she" does not imply the exclusion of any person.

    In an effort to avoid confusion, the author has chosen to conform to the Western custom of placing surnames last rather than first, which is routine in Asia. The only exceptions are General Choi Hang Hi and General Kim Yu Shin, since they are universally recognized by this iteration.

Dedication

This book is dedicated to my teacher Grandmaster Richard Chun. For his wisdom, support and, above all, his patience.

Contents

Contents

Foreword

Grandmaster Richard Chun

So much about taekwondo has changed since the 1960s when I began teaching in New York City. Back then the term taekwondo was seldom used by schools to describe the style they featured, favoring instead to advertise as karate academies, an imprimatur more familiar to the public in general. While it is considered the most popular martial art in the world today, taekwondo had not yet found its identity as an Olympic sport and the various institutes or *kwans* had only recently combined under a single standard. Korea, my native land, was still on the mend following the bloody civil conflict of the early 1950s that claimed the lives of so many.

Yet even then I had a clear understanding of where I intended to take the art I had worked so hard to master from an early age. Rather than concentrate purely on the combat sport taekwondo was quickly becoming, I chose instead to promote many of the offensive and defensive skills transmitted to me at the famed Moo Duk Kwan in Seoul by Master Chong Soo Hong. Traditional hand techniques, sweeps, joint locks, and throws were then perceived as being far too dangerous for competition and were subsequently forbidden in the ring. The performance of *poomsae*—the formal exercises representing the essence of the art—was being foreshadowed too by the need to develop modern fighting strategies that would ensure competitive domination in the future. What would become of these hard earned, time tested skills? Would they evaporate and be forgotten like so many other customs throughout the world?

It rapidly became apparent that an organization needed to be created that did not stand in opposition to, but acted in accordance with the various entities that were springing up to support taekwondo as an Olympic sport in America. Undoubtedly, this organization would assist with that worthy goal, but would also continue to propagate the traditional and philosophical aspects of the art. Poomsae, basic technique, ritual one-step sparring, meditation, and self-defense drills would receive equal attention to that of competitive sparring. And so in 1980 I founded the United States Taekwondo Association whose mission was then and remains now the promotion of the ancient and evolving art of taekwondo.

The USTA has currently been in existence for over twenty-five years, and during that time I have cultivated many fine instructors capable of assisting me in the promotion of taekwondo as the traditional martial art that it was intended to be. Some became world champions. Still others went on to establish schools of their own here and abroad. Yet one in particular, Master Doug Cook, has chosen not only to teach professionally, but to follow in my footsteps and support the art through the written word. While teaching five classes a day sometimes as often as seven days a week, he has authored two books published by YMAA, a highly respected member of the literary community. *Taekwondo—Ancient Wisdom for the Modern Warrior* and *Traditional Taekwondo—Core Techniques, History, and Philosophy* both focus on the philosophy and techniques unique to the practice of traditional taekwondo rather than its sportive mate. Both have become best-sellers and have inspired thousands of students around the world.

In *Taekwondo—A Path to Excellence*, his third book, Doug Cook has again touched on virtues, principles, and techniques that are certain to fortify the martial artist of the twenty-first century. This book then is of value for all who seek excellence in their daily pursuits. Qualities, such as enduring strength, the doctrine of purpose, and respect for tradition, are as applicable to the martial artist as they are to the ordinary individual looking to navigate the adversities modern life proffers.

Still, it is traditional taekwondo based on an action philosophy that this book primarily addresses, and it gives me great comfort and satisfaction to see one of my senior students carry on the traditions I have espoused for so long. In a world of commercial expediency it is easy to fall victim to greed and compromise. Yet Master Cook has consistently taken the high road in providing his students and his readers with high quality instruction and eminent prose. I commend him for his tireless efforts and highly recommend his books to anyone interested in cultivating an enhanced lifestyle through a diligent practice of the traditional martial arts.

Grandmaster Richard Chun
9th dan black belt
President, United States
Taekwondo Association

Preface

The inspiration for this book first crystallized at thirty-five thousand feet over Arizona one Sunday morning many years ago during a flight to California. A freshly-minted novice at the time, fired with enthusiasm, I would have much preferred to be standing at attention in my taekwondo class that was coincidently just beginning back in New York rather than sitting shoe-horned into an economy seat that seemed to be shrinking by the minute. In a meager act of contrition, I began to read a celebrated work on the martial arts published over a quarter century ago. With chapters no longer than three or four pages in length and print large enough for an adult with failing eyesight to comfortably read, it still holds water to this day. The ability to pick up this modest tome and within the space of a few short minutes receive a complete dose of knowledge in one sitting was satisfying to say the least.

Since then, over the course of my training, I have read many books devoted to an exploration of the martial arts. Some qualify as true purveyors of wisdom; others less so. Nevertheless, I have endeavored on two separate occasions to contribute to the former, the success of which can only be measured by the reader. Beyond that it has been my privilege to craft frequent articles focusing on traditional taekwondo for several noted magazines. This book, my third, while loosely based on a collection of those writings, has been expanded significantly to include philosophical insights based on a doctrine of purpose as taught to me by my teacher, Grandmaster Richard Chun. This book is about a journey whose ultimate destination is the achievement of physical and spiritual enrichment through the disciplined practice of a traditional martial art. Rather than simply plotting formulas certain to score in the ring, I have attempted to impart essential, defensive elements of the art, both physical and intellectual, that conform to the principle of *Do*, or *The Way* of taekwondo. Without this crucial knowledge, practice becomes a peripheral component of existence rather than an organic ingredient supporting a meaningful life.

It is my sincere hope that this book will act as an inspiration to martial artists of all styles, levels, and ages. Although its concentration clearly rests on traditional taekwondo as opposed to its sportive mate, the philosophy within can be applied to all disciplines regardless of heritage. If the reader is driven to train with increased vigor, further investigate his art through prose, or simply enjoy his practice due to an enhanced view of its philosophical underpinnings, then I have accomplished my goal.

Master Doug Cook
5th dan black belt

Acknowledgments

There are many individuals who have graciously contributed to the successful completion of this work. Certain places, too, have provided a peaceful setting conducive to creative writing. Subsequently, I would like to express my deep appreciation and thanks to the following:

Catherine DeCesare for the many illustrations throughout this book aptly depicting the true heart of traditional taekwondo . . . here, she is the Um to my Yang.

Grandmaster Woojin Jung, Carol Davis Hart, and Laura Stolpe of Tri-Mount Publications, publishers of *TaeKwonDo Times* magazine, for providing me with a forum to express my passion for taekwondo through my *Traditions* column.

David Ripianzi, Tim Comrie, and my editor, Barbara Langley, of YMAA Publication Center, for their tireless efforts in making yet another dream come true.

The talented John Jordan III and Henry Smith for their timeless photographic gifts.

Masters Samuel Mizrahi, Pablo Alejandro, Richard Conceicao, and James Vandenburg Jr. for their technical contributions to the Chosun Taekwondo Academy.

Grandmaster Gyoo Hyun Lee and Master Ryan An for providing us with excellent training while in South Korea.

The instructors, students, parents, and friends of the Chosun Taekwondo Academy for their dedication to taekwondo and for their support of our school.

Kristen Ciliberti and Christie Ranieri for giving Warwick, New York *The Tuscan Café*, a nexus for creativity.

Joe Hyams for *Zen in the Martial Arts* . . . an enchanting book that cannot help but inspire.

My mother and father, Roy and Joan Cook, for showing me *The Way* in the first place.

And most importantly, Patricia Ann, Erin Elizabeth, and Kristin Lee Cook for a never-ending universe of love, understanding and encouragement. To whatever Energy governs us, Bless Them.

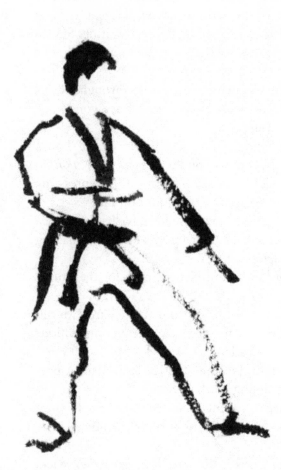

Part One

What Is Taekwondo?

Defining an Art

TAEKWONDO—the traditional martial art and Olympic sport of Korea, an Asian discipline with over sixty-million practitioners worldwide.[1] What is it about this unique way of life targeted at cultivating the mind, body, and spirit that has captured the hearts and minds of so many? Could it be that taekwondo contains over 3,200 empty-hand combat techniques with proven effectiveness on the field of battle establishing it as an authentic means of self-defense?[2] Or is it the metaphysical and philosophical aspects of the art that attract those seeking more than just a simple, physical workout. Perhaps it is the fact that in a constellation of many martial disciplines, taekwondo shares the spotlight, along with judo, as being the only two recognized by the International Olympic Committee IOC and having the exclusive privilege of participating in the Olympic Games. Either way, it is clear that taekwondo has taken its place as the fastest growing, most popular martial art in the world today.

Without a doubt, the current popularity enjoyed by taekwondo, literally translated as "foot-hand-way," or "the way of striking with hands and feet," is largely due to the tireless efforts of several international organizations supported by seasoned master instructors who have dedicated their lives to promoting the art around the globe. Where many martial arts have attempted to attain Olympic recognition and failed, taekwondo has successfully managed to do so through an ingenious process of standardization introduced during its formative years by the Korea Taekwondo Association (KTA), the World Taekwondo Federation (WTF), and the Kukkiwon, center of taekwondo operations worldwide. This development required the core infrastructure of taekwondo to become unified and thus transferable wherever it is taught.

Mirroring its success as a competitive entity, the martial art of taekwondo with roots that date back to antiquity, different from the martial sport bearing the same name, has preserved its technical skills and combat integrity through the efforts of several institutions, including the International Taekwon-Do Federation (ITF) and the United States Taekwondo Association (USTA), organizations that perpetuated taekwondo as a traditional method of self-defense.

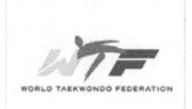 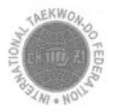

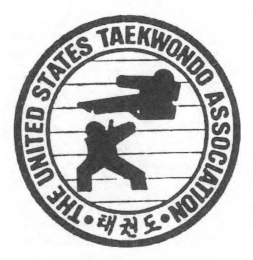

World Taekwondo Federation, International Taekwon-Do Federation, and United States Taekwondo Association emblems.

The WTF, ITF, the Kukkiwon, and the USTA have contributed greatly to the promotion of taekwondo around the world and are virtually responsible for its vast popularity. It is essential that students become acquainted with these organizations in order to appreciate their historical significance and the important role they will play in the future.

On March 22, 1966, taekwondo assumed its rightful place as a global martial art with the founding of the ITF under the direction of General Choi Hong Hi. What began as a group of nine charter nations, including Korea, Malaysia, Vietnam, Singapore, West Germany, America, Egypt, Italy, and Turkey, quickly grew into a worldwide organization boasting over thirty member countries. Viewed as a stronghold of traditional taekwondo technique, the ITF flourished and continues to maintain a strong global presence to this day.

Considered the guardian of sport taekwondo, the WTF was established on June 3, 1973. This organization effectively replaced the ITF following its relocation abroad and is responsible for developing modern, innovative methods of competition while at the same time maintaining traditional technique. As with any complex organization, the WTF is composed of many specialized entities including the financial, women's, collegiate, and referee committees. Its origin followed a meeting of the thirty delegate countries that had participated in the First World Taekwondo Championships held at the Kukkiwon in May of 1973. At this meeting Dr. Un Yong Kim was elected the first president of the new federation. Presently, with its headquarters at the Joyang Building, Seoul, South Korea, the WTF acts as a clearinghouse for tens of thousands of applicants throughout the world seeking legitimate black belt certification through their national governing bodies. Due to the stewardship of its many experienced officials, coupled with its 189 member nations, taekwondo remains the only martial art, other than judo, to maintain official Olympic status.

The USTA, whose mission it is to "promote the ancient and evolving art of taekwondo," was established in 1980 by

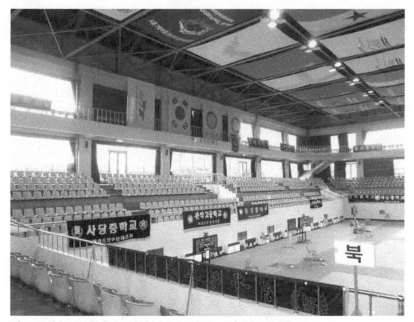

The Kukkiwon, located in Seoul, South Korea.

Grandmaster Richard Chun who continues to serve as its president. Currently, the USTA supports a mix of traditional skills combined with competitive and educational events that reflect the demographics of its membership.

Literally translated as "National Gymnasium," the Kukkiwon is located atop a hillside in the Kangnam District of Seoul. Construction began on November 9, 1971, with the facility being inaugurated on November 30, 1972. Mirroring traditional Korean architecture, its humble exterior is deceptive as it houses management offices, locker rooms, seminar space, and a museum. Practitioners from every corner of the globe visit the Taekwondo Academy housed at the Kukkiwon to take advantage of the comprehensive instructor program available to advanced students. Standing alone on the well-trodden wooden floor of this dynamic monument to taekwondo is an awe-inspiring experience to say the least. Students cannot help but sense the lingering spirit generated by the many dedicated Korean martial artists who have, over the decades, devoted their lives to the refinement of the art.

Yet it is important to note that taekwondo is not merely about kicking and punching. Rather it is an action philosophy that seeks to enrich the lives of those who diligently apply its honorable principles to their daily routine. For decades taekwondo has been the perfect medium for cultivating inner strength, extraordinary endurance, and an effective arsenal of defensive skills. In its current iteration it can be thought of as a reflection of modern society's desire for a ritualized discipline devoid of religious dogma but complete with both a physically and spiritually enhanced set of ethical principles by which to live. This is a result of the art's virtuous foundation influenced by the three Asian philosophical paradigms of Buddhism, Confucianism, and Taoism.[3] Even though these philosophies were never meant to become deified or transformed into religions by their originators, they have over the centuries essentially evolved into just that. However, it is the virtues and principles bundled within these ancient ideologies that the martial artist embraces and not the theology itself. For the sincere practitioner, doctrines borrowed from these systems act as a moral compass in pointing the way toward self-improvement.

Although Taoism is rooted in Chinese culture with a firm basis in non-intervention and pursuit of the one, true path or *The Way*, it has played a significant role in the development of the Korean martial arts. As we shall see, the *poomsae* or formal exercises that stand as a central pillar in the practice of traditional taekwondo reflect the eight aspects of the *I Ching* or *The Classic of Changes* (Korean: *Juyeok*), a cornerstone of Taoism. Taoist *qigong*, too, can be practiced by the taekwondoist as a method of enhancing the body's internal energy or *Ki*.

Confucianism, with its origin steeped in the cultivation of a superior lifestyle through ethical behavior, supplies us with the code of honor Korean stylists strive to live by. *The Five Tenets of Taekwondo*—Courtesy, Integrity, Perseverance, Self-Control, and Indomitable Spirit—come to us not only as a gift from General

Choi Hong Hi, an important figure in the establishment of tae-kwondo, but also from the Confucian-based segment of the Asian philosophical triad.

Yet perhaps the most obvious manifestation of Confucian-ism is exemplified in the system of seniority we find not only in the martial arts, but in Asian culture in general. For example, it is not unusual in Korea for its citizens to expend much energy in the service of a senior regardless of whether the level of re-spect is contingent upon a chronological or academic standard. In taekwondo this hierarchal structure is clearly evident in the student/teacher relationship and through the courtesy afforded senior belts by juniors.

While Buddhism, likely considered the most generous con-tributor to the Korean martial arts, took a back seat to Confu-cianism during the Chosun Dynasty (A.D. 1392-1910), in Korea today it continues to remain one of the leading spiritual pursuits, along with Christianity.[4] According to legend, it was the Bud-dhist patriarch Bodhidharma who created a component of the Chinese fighting arts from which taekwondo has drawn much of its soft or circular movements. Buddhist doctrine, as handed down in the seventh-century by the venerable Buddhist monk Wonkwang Popsa, established a code of ethics against which the *Hwarang* warriors of the Silla Dynasty (57 B.C.–A.D. 935) fought for unification of the Three Kingdoms. As if these contributions were not enough, *Zen* (Korean: *Sun*) Buddhism modeled a means for devotees and martial artists alike to calm the mind through the practice of seated meditation or *zazen*, developed by the Zen monk Dogen in A.D. 1253.

But taekwondo is first and foremost an *action* philosophy and as such must be *physically* practiced. Regardless of the philo-sophical contributions of the past, taekwondo is very much like an apple; we can speak about its genus, color, and texture, but until we take a bite, chew it, taste it, and swallow it, we will never really know what an apple is all about. The same holds true with our practice. It is essential to view taekwondo from a historical and philosophical perspective, but just as necessary

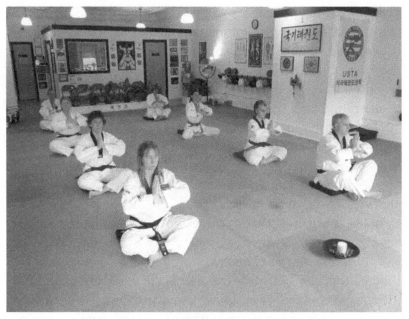

Martial artists embrace meditation as a method of quieting the mind prior to intense training.

to seek excellence in physical technique. Understanding the importance of this concept, let us explore the elements that qualify taekwondo as a traditional, combat-proven martial art.

The Vital Elements of Taekwondo: The Three-Legged Stool

The art of taekwondo can be viewed as a vast mosaic composed of diverse components that, taken together, form a comprehensive system of self-defense, physical fitness, and spiritual enrichment. Ignoring any one of these components will lead to weakness in the others. This synergy brings to mind an observation I once made during the early years of my training.

One spring day while out driving, I took notice of what looked to be a perfectly good stool standing askew at the end of someone's driveway next to the trash cans. Upon closer inspection, I

7

realized that one of its three legs was missing, essentially rendering it useless. It dawned on me that an allegory could be drawn between this damaged piece of furniture in need of repair and the vital elements that comprise the core curriculum of traditional taekwondo. Here's how I arrived at this seemingly odd connection.

In his inspiring video *Budo Sai: The Spirit of the Samurai*, British *karateka* Terry O'Neill affirms the importance of three fundamentals that are common to all classical martial arts. In the case of *Shotokan karate-do*, these elements are *kihon, kata,* and *kumite*, or, as O'Neill suggests, the "three K's." Being the complete martial art that it is, taekwondo is not immune to this principle. It, too, is composed of three crucial components. The Korean terms for these, however, are *kibon, poomsae,* and *kyorugi*. In both cases, literally translated, the three terms can be defined respectively as basics, forms, and sparring. These elements represent the foundation upon which any traditional martial art sits. Clearly, any serious pursuit of taekwondo demands that the practitioner become proficient in the rudiments of the art. Deficiency in any one of the above will cause the student to falter overall since all three are interdependent. Therefore, the analogy surfaces that just as a stool requires three legs to stand upright so the taekwondoist must cultivate basic skills, meaningful forms, and effective sparring in order to have both feet firmly planted in the art.

The First Leg: Kibon/Basics

Taken individually, *basics*, the first element or leg in the triad of traditional training, provides the practitioner with a solid base composed of the individual tools necessary to define movement as effective defensive and offensive strategy. Foremost in this category, along with an understanding of Korean history and culture, is a working knowledge of rooted stances, powerful blocks, numerous hand strikes, footwork, kicks with proper trajectory, and an application of body mechanics. When practicing in Korea, my students and I are often required to throw a kick hundreds of times or hold a stance for many minutes while the headmaster tests the angle of our hands, arms, legs, and feet. Intense training of this nature frequently goes on for hours and allows us to mindfully monitor all aspects of body alignment, forcing forgetful muscles to remember details that will resurface time and time again in the future. For the black belt, reviewing basic technique alongside the novice is never a chore but an exercise in renewal. With each middle strike, low block, or front kick, the body learns to organize energy equally in both the right and left sides, increase focus, project strength, and maintain balance.

Securing a practical understanding of the Korean language, coupled with an appreciation for the culture that spawned taekwondo, adds color and vitality to concerted practice. As a case in point, words are symbols that conjure up images in our mind causing physiological responses that result in specific actions. Subsequently, using two disparate terms for the same subject may produce contrasting mental images. For example, the Korean command, *"dwiro dora,"* stoutly said, summons up an entirely different image in our consciousness than would simply shouting "about face." The former pronouncement is ripe with

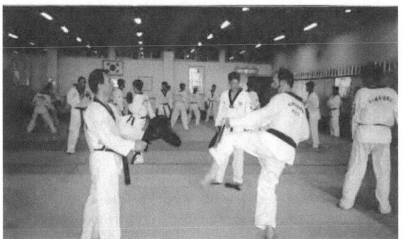

Photo by John Jordan III

Kicking drills at the Korean National University for Physical Education in Seoul, South Korea.

the phonetics and spirit unique to the Korean language and may produce a motion more precise than that elicited by its English counterpart. Classical ballet, a discipline remarkably similar in body mechanics to traditional taekwondo, unfailingly subscribes to this practice in its use of French terminology. Think of it; a wizened dance master directing her students to "spin around," rather than "pirouette," would in all likelihood be ushered off the floor of the dance studio in disgrace!

Although decidedly academic rather than physical in nature, developing an objective viewpoint of Korean history creates a chronological and geographical connection with the people and places that profoundly influenced traditional taekwondo during its formative years. Without this perspective it is difficult for the practitioner to fully comprehend the passions that drove the Korean people to create such an art in the first place. It should be realized that the drama and dignity that accentuated the evolution of taekwondo represented, in some ways, a microcosm of Korean culture in general during the chaotic 1940s and 50s. It is difficult for us today to fully comprehend the death and destruction that accompanied the civil strife resulting from the Japanese Occupation, World War II, and the Korean Conflict. Seoul, the capital city, was decimated under a merciless rain of bombs originating from friend and foe alike with its citizenry scurrying to every corner of Asia for safe haven.[5] Its infrastructure resembled the picked over carcass of some long-deceased animal; its bridges were twisted heaps of metal, its buildings skeletal shadows of their former selves. Orphans scavenged through mountains of trash for any morsel of nutrition to be found.[6] Hope in life hung by a gossamer thread. Yet the tenacity and vision of the Korean people—in spite of *han,* the chronic sorrow ingrained within the national psyche multiplied by centuries of adversity—prevailed in their desire to resurrect a golden past wrapped in honor. Through great effort, the strategically-significant peninsula was revitalized into a thriving industrial power, although one that today remains divided by a fundamental ideology. Likewise, Korean martial artists were splintered in their own way by dissimilar styles, an infiltration of foreign influences, and a strong nationalistic desire to shake off the yoke of Japanese rule. Passions ran high with master instructors and heads of institutes attempting to distance themselves from a reliance on Chinese and Japanese martial disciplines in an effort to shore up their own native styles.[7] Yet perhaps unknowingly at the time, the Korean martial art was poised for a catharsis in its rally for world recognition. Profound decisions would be made by prominent players in government and the military, with paths being plotted that would eventually lead the ravaged nation through its martial arts heritage to Olympic gold. This turbulent historical record cannot be ignored if the taekwondo student wishes to absorb the art in its entirety.[8] Knowledge of these significant events is as important as the proper basic execution of a side kick, knife hand block, or middle strike.

The Second Leg: Poomsae/Forms

Poomsae, or forms, the second key component of the taekwondo syllabus, represent a common denominator within all classical martial arts. Also known as *hyung* (category) or *tul* (pattern), formal exercises symbolize the lifeblood of traditional taekwondo. Poomsae can be defined as choreographed techniques, rich with martial intent, aimed at defeating multiple attackers coming from different directions. They provide the art with character and define its objectives. Forms practice challenges those who persevere through the belt ranks and supplies a vehicle for venerable masters to transmit timeless and often hidden skills to loyal students. It should be pointed out that, in years past, the bulk of martial arts training was handed down through the practice of the formal exercises. Sport-sparring was rare or virtually nonexistent; if the martial artist fought at all, it was for self-preservation.

Since forms are performed in solo fashion, poomsae can be practiced anywhere, anytime. Across the centuries, Asian martial artists have taken advantage of nature, practicing poomsae in densely wooded forests or high in the mountains. Furthermore, forms can be viewed as a catalog of techniques that have been developed over time to take advantage of an ethnic body style

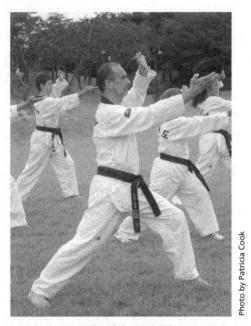

Photo by Patricia Cook

Poomsae represent the method by which martial arts skills were handed down from master to disciple over the centuries.

frequently dictated by the geography and the mindset of a nation. It is said that the topography of a region determines the martial style favored by its local citizenry. As a historical generality, tribes at home on the plains tended to develop equestrian skills, leaving the upper body free to cultivate empty-hand striking techniques coupled with expertise in archery and swordsmanship. On the other hand, warriors trained in predominantly mountainous areas tended to favor defensive skills requiring strong leg muscles, resulting in powerful kicking techniques. Justifiably, the formal defensive patterns exclusive to a particular culture would reflect these idiosyncrasies.

It is extremely important to note that poomsae practice not only embodies, along with sparring, the primary physical element of traditional taekwondo, but a highly spiritual component as well. To appreciate the essence of this concept, we must journey back to ancient times.

It is said that almost five thousand years ago the Taoist sage *Fu Hsi* (2953-2838 B.C.) composed the *I Ching,* considered by many, in conjunction with the *Tao Te Ching* or *The Classic Way of Virtue,* to be the basis of Taoist philosophy.[9] This canon, later amended by Confucius (551-479 B.C.), acted as an oracle for those seeking advice in business, politics, military affairs, and daily life in general. The formula for use of this system supporting the inevitability of change is largely based upon the *duality of opposites* or the *Yin/Yang* (Korean: *Um/Yang*). A popular illustration depicts the Yin/Yang surrounded by eight trigrams composed of solid and broken lines. This symbol is universally known in Korea as the *Palgwe.* Subsequently, these eight aspects combine to create sixty-four hexagrams providing the final tools, along with the casting of yarrow stalks or three Chinese coins, necessary to manipulate the *I Ching.*

Not surprisingly, given the influence of Taoism on traditional taekwondo, a direct correlation exists between the eight original trigrams symbolizing heaven, lake, fire, thunder, wind, water, mountain, and earth, and the philosophical concepts that underscore the eight *Taegeuk* and Palgwe poomsae currently sanctioned by the WTF. Since the Taegeuk and Palgwe series appear in sets, the individual poomsae can be thought of as chapters of a book, each signifying a unique philosophy. For example, *Taegeuk Yook Jang,* whose *I Ching* component is a broken line over a solid line with another broken line beneath, symbolizes water and focuses on our ability to overcome life's adversities by exhibiting the patience, consistency, and flow of a great river. Likewise, poomsae *Taegeuk Chil Jang* is signified by two broken lines below a single, solid line. The philosophical principle of this poomsae is *mountain* and teaches the practitioner when to advance and when to hesitate, mirroring the behavior of an experienced climber as he progressively attains the summit. Additionally, all nine WTF black belt poomsae, or *Yudanja* forms, are steeped in traditional principles ranging from *Koryo,* a pattern demonstrating strength as expressed through conviction, to poomsae *Ilyo,* representing the Buddhist quest for oneness or nirvana.[10]

Poomsae Philosophical Concepts
and their
Relationship to the Eight Trigrams of the I Ching

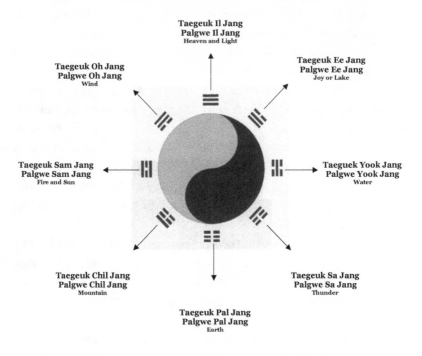

Taegeuk Il Jang
Palgwe Il Jang
Heaven and Light

Taegeuk Ee Jang
Palgwe Ee Jang
Joy or Lake

Taegeuk Oh Jang
Palgwe Oh Jang
Wind

Taegeuk Sam Jang
Palgwe Sam Jang
Fire and Sun

Taeguek Yook Jang
Palgwe Yook Jang
Water

Taegeuk Chil Jang
Palgwe Chil Jang
Mountain

Taegeuk Sa Jang
Palgwe Sa Jang
Thunder

Taegeuk Pal Jang
Palgwe Pal Jang
Earth

A discreet set of ideals, in many cases tied to personalities and events in Korean history, are assigned to the ITF patterns or tul created by General Choi Hong Hi. By way of example, the second tul in the series of twenty-four known as the *Chang-Han* (Blue Cottage) series memorializes *Tangoon* (ca. 2333 B.C.), the mythical progenitor of Korea, while the last, *Tong Il*, represents the future unification of the nation which was divided, North and South, in 1945 and unfortunately remains so today.

It is sometimes claimed that the connection of a philosophical component with the physical practice of poomsae is at best a stretch of the imagination. However, this pairing presents a treasure trove for those of us seeking more than an aerobic workout from our training. Simply because taekwondo, with roots dating back to antiquity, was officially established in the 1950s, does not mean it cannot share in ancient philosophical paradigms embraced by Asian culture as a whole. Korean society was greatly influenced by Buddhist and Confucian doctrine during the reign of the Silla, Koryo, and Chosun dynasties. So why then should its native martial art not respectfully reflect this legacy in some way? Granted, Taoism played the least significant role in molding the nation's character. Yet even the South Korean flag, with the Um/Yang and its four trigrams, bears witness to the important contribution the *I Ching* and Taoism have had on the collective consciousness of the Korean people.

Today, schools featuring mixed, non-traditional martial arts have chosen to ignore the importance of the archetypal, formal exercises coupled with their philosophical foundation. If practiced at all, forms are often relegated to a position equal to that of warm-up exercises. Regretfully, even the late Bruce Lee was heard to say that poomsae training is tantamount to "learning to swim on dry land." Still, metaphorically speaking, a contemporary painter applies brushstrokes from a palette of colors that have existed from time immemorial to create a canvas washed in art. What then is to preclude a modern martial artist from using ancient philosophical symbols to embellish his art?

Rigorous poomsae training permits the martial artist to string together individual techniques gleaned from a diligent practice of basics into sequences of effective defensive tactics and counterattacks. It provides a method for cultivating stamina, focus, balance, and agility. Finally, the dynamic movements of poomsae, though pre-arranged, act as a bridge to step-sparring, sophisticated self-defense tactics, and ultimately free-sparring.

The Third Leg: Kyorugi/Sparring

The third essential piece of the puzzle in the traditional taekwondo curriculum, kyorugi, or sparring, represents a collection of ritualized offensive and defensive scenarios unique to many hard-style martial arts. These include *il su sik* (one-step sparring), *ee su sik* (two-step sparring), *sam su sik* (three-step sparring), and *machueo kyorugi* (pre-arranged sparring). Free sparring will take into account traditional point sparring and WTF Olympic-style sparring. Although limited to various grabs, release, and joint locking techniques, *ho sin sool* (self-defense skills) will be examined as well. Often ho sin sool techniques will be combined with il su sik in a pre-arranged fashion defined as *ho sin sool kyorugi* (self-defense sparring).

Taken as a whole, the practice of il su sik, ee su sik, and sam su sik may at first appear artificial in nature by virtue of its choreographed precision, but as a practical method of self-defense training, it serves a variety of purposes. Primarily, this ritualized form of practice allows the student to launch predetermined defensive tactics against an opponent, confident that there will be little danger of injury. Since there is seldom any hard contact made, practitioners of all ages and both genders can benefit from this form of training. The term "one-step sparring" is so named because the aggressor advances one step forward while attacking, prior to the defender initiating an appropriate defense. The drill consists of two students facing one another at a minimum distance of three feet with a maximum distance not to exceed the height of the taller participant. One of the pair, being assigned the role of attacker, will step back with the right leg into a front stance while simultaneously executing a left low block and a *kihop*. The defender will then yell "kihop," signaling his preparedness to defend. The aggressor, advancing one step forward, then executes a predetermined strike punctuated again by a firm "kihop." Consequently, the defending student will mount an appropriate defense counterbalanced by a counter-attack commensurate with his level of proficiency. One-step sparring strategy, for the most part, prepares the student to defend against the lunge punch, perhaps the most prevalent offensive tool common to nearly all confrontations. This by no means excludes defense against other related instruments of attack, such as the front kick or round kick.

Aside from one-step sparring, the taekwondoist also practices two and three-step sparring. These training scenarios differ from il su sik in that the designated attacker, rather than advancing

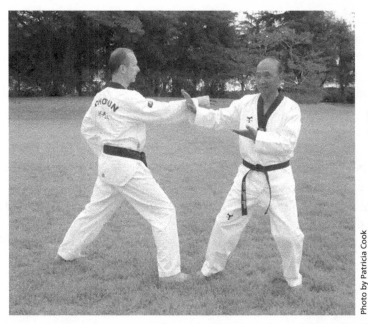

Photo by Patricia Cook

Step sparring represents a safe and effective way to practice defensive strategies against various strikes and kicks. Here, Grandmaster Richard Chun demonstrates a technique with the author while training in Korea.

one step, advances two or three steps while mounting a pre-determined attack. In the case of the novice, the attacking technique can be the same, for example, three high punches in consecutive order. When practiced by the advanced student, a combination of challenging techniques may be used instead.

Additionally, ho sin sool or self-defense techniques provide solutions against various grabs including, but not exclusive to, headlocks, bear hugs, full and half nelsons, cross hand grabs, shoulder grabs, and same side grabs. Weapon defense, too, plays an important role in ho sin sool practice. Many of the concepts involved in ho sin sool are based on the concept of redirecting an aggressor's negative Ki during an attack, causing it to betray him in the process. Many of these skills are derived from the Korean martial art of *hapkido* or "the way of harmonizing Ki."[11]

Prearranged sparring represents another method of self-defense training. Here partners are again alternately assigned the roles of attacker and defender, each utilizing a series of favored techniques that complement body style and proficiency. This is not yet considered free-sparring since one partner is defending by stepping back and blocking while the other is attacking in a free-style manner.

Free-sparring permits two students who are facing one another to engage in a form of practice where both are attacking and defending simultaneously based on opportunity. An opening in one student's defensive strategy is exploited by the other and vice versa. Even though free-sparring mirrors real-life fighting conditions, it is still constrained by the rules of the game and the use of required safety gear. In the case of traditional point-sparring, participants generally wear foam head, hand, and foot

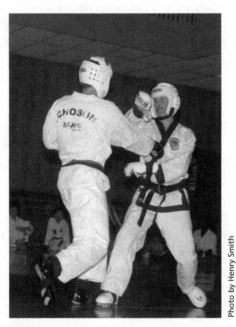

Photo by Henry Smith

Prearranged and free-sparring permits the martial artist to express advanced skills in a unique manner while becoming aware of strengths and weaknesses.

protectors. Contact is often limited in power and the match is stopped following a successful strike at which time the referee awards the appropriate points. In WTF Olympic-style sparring, perhaps the most popular form of sparring in taekwondo today, competitors don fabric forearm guards along with shin/instep protectors, foam helmets, and chest protectors or *hogu*. There is no halt to the action between points with full contact permitted resulting in body displacement. Points are awarded during the match through electronic means, or manually at its completion.

Coupled with the use of innovative safety equipment, free-sparring teaches the student how to convert a threatening situation to his advantage through the use of superior strategy and a strong will. Naturally, in today's sport-oriented society, sparring is often used as a means of competition and entertainment. Free-sparring further represents a decisive means for individual expression of the art in conjunction with a ritualized collection of defensive and offensive strategies. Unlimited possibilities exist when combining techniques in answer to an opponent's measured attack; strengths and weaknesses are amplified, bringing a winning score to the former and a painful lesson in the case of the latter. A ruffian off the street can throw a flurry of wild punches. But in the ring and on the training hall floor, only an accomplished martial artist can demonstrate the consistency, flow, breath control, and raw power required to deliver well-placed kicks and hand strikes, as in the case of point-sparring, within inches of an opponent's vital points. Then, should it ultimately become necessary due to an escalation of aggression beyond verbal mediation, that minor gap in space can be closed quickly with one strike confidently concluding the altercation.

Were it not for the ritualized practice of il su sik, ee su sik, sam su sik, ho sin sool, and kyorugi, traditional taekwondo practice could potentially evolve into a chaotic and painful pursuit. Most martial artists, due to the very nature of their art, learn to accept a modicum of discomfort in the course of their training. However, this does not mean that they take pleasure from it nor does it exempt them from injury. The serious practitioner of traditional taekwondo, by using such training strategies, will continue to develop an understanding of safety, courtesy, distancing, power, body mechanics, breath control, use of Ki, and presence of mind, culminating in a deep appreciation for the true essence of martial arts doctrine.

But our analogy of a three-legged stool does not end with the vital elements that authenticate the holistic nature of traditional taekwondo. Aside from the physical manifestation of the art, the student strives to cultivate a strong character supported by an enlightened mind. The martial artist's disposition is strengthened by nurturing indomitable will and patience while the spirit is enhanced through Ki development exercises and meditation. Though metaphysical in appearance, the synergy created by the magnification of mind, body, and spirit symbolizes the maturation and fulfillment of the practitioner. And here, again, the number three is significant.

Surprisingly, even the philosophy that underscores the design of the *dobok*, the V-neck style uniform worn by the taekwondoist, flirts with the power of three. Information provided by the KTA introduces the notion that this training garment is inspired by the *hanbok*—the traditional clothing worn by native Koreans for centuries. Particular attention is given to three distinct shapes that comprise the dobok. The waistline conforms to a circle, the hip area describes a triangle, and the cuffs trace a square. The top of the dobok is constructed in the same manner. The three geometric designs denote heaven (*won*-circle), earth (*bang*-triangle), and mankind (*kak*-square) respectively.[12] Taken as a whole, these three symbols represent the foundation of our universe (*samsilshingo*).[13]

Similarly, it is rare when traveling in Korea to see the blue and red taegeuk (Um/Yang) as a standalone icon except as an imprint on the Korean flag. Instead, a symbol characterized as the *samgeuk* abounds on any number of cultural items from ancient drum heads to modern marketing products. The samgeuk is a circle composed of the colors red, blue, and yellow, spiraling inward signifying the harmonizing coexistence of heaven, earth, and humankind.

Certainly, a close examination of any traditional martial art will reveal peripheral aspects that do not fit easily into the three categories described above. Breaking, or *kyuk pa*, an additional element of taekwondo as pointed out in the *Kukkiwon Textbook*, is an important vehicle in testing the raw power of any strike.[14] Impractical as it would be to assess our skill utilizing full force on an unprotected human target, the breaking of a solid object such as wood or a brick permits the practitioner to gauge penetrating force in a meaningful way. Without a doubt, breaking, at least in the eyes of the general public, represents the most dramatic demonstration of martial arts technique!

Ki development is another essential ingredient of martial arts training that is often ignored and may be due to the metaphysical issues it raises. Yet teaching traditional taekwondo without offering the practitioner exercises in Ki development is tantamount

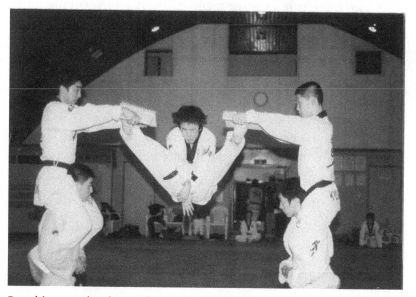

Breaking, or kyuk pa, dramatically demonstrates the penetrating power of taekwondo through indomitable will.

to sitting someone behind the steering wheel of a car, but telling them nothing of the fuel that powers its engine. Ki is the elixir that amplifies technique and triggers great strength; it is the force that shields the body from harm while maintaining health and a sense of well being. Grandmaster Richard Chun, a true pioneer and practitioner of traditional taekwondo, states that "Ki is the cosmic ocean in which everything exists."[15] Likewise, William Reed, a disciple of Koichi Tohei, founder of *Shin Shin Totsu Aikido*, describes Ki as "a universal energy capable of infinite expansion and contraction, which can be directed, but not contained, by the mind."[16] Today, the relevance of Ki is appreciated by millions of people around the world. Those who practice qigong do so in order to nurture health and a greater sense of well being. Still, the full understanding of this vital life force remains a mystery in no small part due to its evanescent nature. Even though martial arts students in general have great faith in Ki, studies have been conducted in an attempt to confirm its reality. But at present, even though energy fields surrounding the body have been measured, no concrete clinical evidence is available to support its existence.

Clearly, the rule of three seems to exert an overriding influence on all aspects of traditional taekwondo. And just as a three-legged stool with one defective leg will cease to support weight and ultimately become useless, our technique will suffer significantly should we ignore the importance of kibon, poomsae, and kyorugi. Do not wind up at the end of the training driveway next to the trash cans of discarded martial arts techniques. To benefit greatly, continuously and with diligence apply the final application of the number three in taekwondo . . . *practice, practice, practice*!

The Importance of *Do*

The term taekwondo is composed of three simple syllables representing a universe of power. Certainly, the consequences of striking with feet, *tae*, and fists, *kwon*, are clear. However, to underestimate the significance of the last syllable, *do*, due to its grammatical positioning within the root word taekwondo, is to admit to a profound ignorance in this diverse, holistic discipline. To subtract this suffix entirely is to remove the heart and soul of the art, transforming it instead into a mere pugilistic pursuit, a hollow, physical exercise rather than an organic philosophy complete with a ritualized set of moral principles.

Pronounced "doe," this elegant two-character syllable above all symbolizes the spiritual, intellectual, and ethical dimensions manifest in the traditional Korean martial art of taekwondo. Literally translated, *do* is *The Way* or path every martial artist must travel. It is the essence and standard against which all practical and theoretical technique is measured. It is the level we must seek, the ideal we embrace. It is a continuum the sincere practitioner will visit time and time again with never any hope of reaching an end. It is a work constantly in progress. Grandmaster Sang Kyu Shim put this journey into perspective when he wrote: "One must not confuse the skills of living with *The Way* of living. The martial arts point the way while providing the skills to follow *The Way*. This is the road to creative change, a road of encounter and discovery. It is the road of a million miles that begins with the first step."[17]

The contemporary model of *do* primarily stems from a desire expressed by noted masters of the past to transform their traditional fighting skills, no longer as relevant in times of peace, into martial *ways*. Simply put, a martial *way* distinguishes itself from a battle art in that the ultimate goal is not necessarily one of combat preparedness so much as it is in discovering a method or means to achieve personal excellence through a practice of the martial arts accompanied by their implied codes of honor. By way of example, taekwondo, tangsoodo, karate-do, aikido, and judo are all offspring of defensive methods whose sole purpose is to subdue an aggressor bent on mortal harm, with little or no regard given to character development. These potent fighting systems, systems such as Japanese *Daito ryu Aiki Jujutsu*, were diluted or sanitized just enough to remain faithful to their original nature but made sufficiently safe for training on a consistent basis by the general public. Men, such as General Choi Hong Hi, Hwang Kee, Yasutsune Itosu, Gichen Funakoshi, Morihei Ueshiba, and Jigoro Kano, appreciated the value of elevating their defensive skills—already steeped in ancient, orthodox philosophies—to vital disciplines intended to instill defensive strategy, confidence, and morality into society at large. Consequently, tens of millions of practitioners worldwide study some form of martial art in an effort to fortify their physical, mental, and spiritual well being while becoming proficient in a form of self-defense. Practitioners of traditional taekwondo further support this model by striving to live a balanced life through a practice of the *Five Tenets*—the virtues the Korean citizenry at large have relied upon, particularly during the twentieth century, in rising from the ashes of war to their present state of economic and cultural development. Taekwondo, being a product of this will to survive coupled with a need to reaffirm a national identity on the heels of Japanese Occupation, has served as a platform for the cultivation of *do*. While it is true that the term taekwondo itself is only a few short decades old, having been coined on April 11, 1955, by General Choi Hong Hi, the fact remains that the *do*, or martial way that we are presently familiar with, resonates with philosophical overtones culled from a mixture of traditional fighting styles and individuals rooted deep in Korean history. We cannot help but appreciate this heritage while visiting the universities, training halls, temples, and monuments built to memorialize these legendary arts and figures. Still, there are those today who assert that taekwondo has no true legacy, that it is nothing more than a competitive sport, a bastard child of Japanese *karate* or Chinese *gungfu*. Forgotten are the centuries of invasion and imperialism during which the Korean people had to defend the sovereignty of their tiny nation with the blood of their young warriors while nurturing a robust code of honor in the process. This courage is evident in every technique of the national Korean martial art.

Taking a utilitarian approach to the basic theme underscoring *The Way* can have a profound effect on the practical application of traditional taekwondo technique in general. For example, the very basis of the martial arts movement, now and in the past, can be traced to the observation and mimicry of nature. The taekwondoist must concede that nature is embraced by *do*. Many of the more advanced strikes and stances, including tiger mouth (*akum sohn*) and cat stance (*bom sogi*), derive their very names from the defensive tactics seen in the animal kingdom. The method of wrist rotation found in the execution of the middle punch (*momtong jiluki*) while in horse stance (*ja choom sogi*) replicates the revolution of the planets as described in the principles of celestial mechanics—a truly grand manifestation of *The Way*.

Taegeuk, Palgwe, and Yudanja poomsae, the formal exercises unique to taekwondo, are rich in an abundance of natural metaphor. With philosophical underpinnings borrowing heavily from the ancient Asian classic, the *I Ching*, the performance of forms represents nature in its fullness. Through a mutual combination of nature and motion coupled with dynamic meditation, the practitioner, over years, learns to overcome the physical limitations of the body, instead experiencing the spiritual aspects of *The Way*.

Natural harmony, too, should be evident in the execution of all techniques as it applies to the human anatomy. By practicing within the constraints of the body's natural range of motion, stress and injury will be brought to a minimum. Permitting the muscles to remain in a relaxed and natural state will result in the development of explosive power upon impact. Consequently, since *The Way* is all-encompassing in its relationship to physiology, natural movement equates to *do*. Clearly, from the early stages of social development on up to the present, an understanding of *do* has been accompanied by a deep appreciation of nature. In fact, one cannot exist without the other.

The Way, then, is unmistakably paved by virtuous thought and action. It is arrived at through diligent practice and a never-ending commitment to excellence. To waver is an admission of one's humanity; to reclaim the rightful path, however, is a definitive sign of discipline and commitment. In the words of the Zen patriarch, Bodhidharma, "All know *The Way*—few actually walk it."

As we advance in the martial arts, a sense of balance, both physically and spiritually, begins to increase. Better health ensues. Reflexes are sharpened and a profound appreciation for the value of life pervades our being. Finally, we are rewarded with increased confidence and self-respect through our knowledge of self-defense. This course is a journey marked by many mileposts. It is a highway whose unbroken line leads to the philosophical and spiritual refinement of the individual. With each new revelation the practitioner comes closer to the ultimate goal of enlightenment. This journey, this road, is called taekwondo and it is defined by its simple, two letter suffix, *do*.

Articulating Martial Art

Since traditional taekwondo is an authentic martial art—the operative word here being *art*—it allows for personal expression within the confines of technical integrity. Many opportunities exist to fulfill humanity's innate desire for spiritual gratification through artistic endeavor. But where do we turn to allow this stream of consciousness to materialize? One obvious place to start is with the performance of poomsae. I recall attending a black belt promotion test once where four candidates were required to demonstrate *Kang Sang Koon,* an intricate 5th dan form. Due to a disparity in physical stature, differences in body dynamics, depth of stances, and height of kicks quickly became apparent. Each executed the poomsae with technical precision, yet all four practitioners clearly exhibited a component of individuality unique to their body style. Inspiring to watch, their performances were truly art in motion.

Personal articulation can also be expressed during free sparring. Figuratively, the blocks, strikes, and kicks found in taekwondo can be thought of as words that compose a sentence. How these words are strung together determines an author's creativity and, clearly, the larger the vocabulary the more colorful the prose. Likewise, black belts proficient in a multitude of techniques ranging from a simple front kick to aerial spinning kicks possess skill sets capable of expressing almost limitless combinations of defensive measures. These advanced movements, in certain non-competitive settings, can be construed as dance because of the grace, balance, and agility required to perform them.

Used as a vehicle for aesthetic articulation, taekwondo is further enhanced by the fact that it is today a martial way rather than a purely pugilistic system exclusively designed to destroy an attacker in combat. Granted, *kongsoodo* (empty-hand-way), and *tangsoodo* (China-hand-way)—both precursors of taekwondo— were introduced to the Korean armed forces through the Oh Do Kwan (Institute of My Way) in 1953 by General Choi Hong Hi, creator of the 29th Infantry Division. Symbolized by an insignia depicting a fist over the Korean peninsula, the "Fist" or *"Il Keu"* Division distinguished itself by merging regulation drills with martial arts training making it a truly unique entity within the Korean military. Yet the vast majority of taekwondo practitioners then and now were not soldiers, but civilians—ordinary human beings for whom injury meant loss of work or a prolonged absence from educational activities. For these individuals, being on the business end of a well-placed back fist no doubt meant severe injury. Similarly, a wrist lock performed with determination could hamper simple dexterous ability for extended periods of time. These techniques are the essence of any defensive martial strategy, begging the practitioner to invariably ask how often they will actually need to utilize these skills in daily life. This is a question worthy of serious consideration pondered by many in the martial arts community to this day.

Paradoxically, individuals who routinely practice a traditional martial art in modern society do so for a myriad of reasons other than to inflict injury on another human being. These reasons can range anywhere from engaging in a decidedly Eastern experience to maintaining physical fitness and instilling focus in children who might otherwise be glued to a television or computer screen. To many adults, who comprise a significant percentage of the current taekwondo population, simply exercising at a gym can be a mind-numbing proposition. Likewise seeking solace in sedentary quests for enlightenment ignores the body's need to articulate itself in the spatial plain. Furthermore, adolescents frequently forced by eager parents to participate in contests of physical superiority on the gaming fields suffer encounters that can prove disheartening at best. Since traditional taekwondo is a comprehensive *art* or *way*, replete with virtue, discipline, and vigorous motion, it has the ability, if taught with passion and sincerity, to fill the vacuum created by the exclusive practice of competitive sport or the dogmatic pursuit of confounding philosophical paradigms.

In his delightfully entertaining book *Iron and Silk*, author and martial artist Mark Salzman attempts to make sense of the enormous time and effort he invests in his *wushu* training. One day, accompanied by his teacher, he visits a Taoist temple high in the mountains of China. There he witnesses a group of young women performing a traditional dance while waving silk handkerchiefs in their hands. Later, upon completing his *taijiquan* session, he questions Teacher Hei about the need for such perseverance in the martial arts since he had never been engaged in a fight nor did he consider himself a fighter. Teacher Hei responds by saying that if he were truly training for combat he would become a soldier. He further points out that the long spear they are wielding has degraded into nothing more than a cultural artifact with no practical value to the modern warrior. Yet he reminded Salzman that it would be tragic to squander skills accumulated over centuries by masters of the art simply in the name of expediency. "I guess I see what you mean," Salzman allows, "but still, what reason can I give myself for all this effort?" Shrugging his shoulders, his teacher admits, "I don't know—why dance with handkerchiefs?"[18]

I am an avid believer in the practical, realistic application of traditional taekwondo technique during the performance of poomsae, when executing basics and while sparring in the ring. If the serious student is to embrace taekwondo in its fullness, an appreciation for precise motion, body placement, and personal expression within the boundaries of technical integrity as it corresponds to the *art* of taekwondo are all essential ingredients of holistic training. Admittedly, even on today's electronic battlefield filled with exotic firearms and tactical weapons, empty-hand combat techniques can prove useful in tight, urban warfare. The majority of our civilian population will hopefully never experience the dangers of hand-to-hand combat. Personally, I practice traditional taekwondo for its inherent defensive aspects coupled with the moral and physical stamina it evokes. But, like many of us, the more I practice, the more I realize I have less to defend against. Not surprisingly, over the course of time constant daily drilling has evolved into a Zen-like state of moving meditation. More and more I find myself performing blocks, kicks, and strikes simply for the *art* of it. Is this wrong? Should I and others like me ultimately be practicing ballet or some other form of artistic dance instead? I think not. Certainly there is a fiercely practical component to our training, but practicality must be, according to the Um/Yang, that ancient icon depicting harmony between opposites, balanced by impracticality, and frankly, art is often impractical. Think of Jackson Pollock, Martha Graham, and, yes, even traditional Chinese performers waving silk handkerchiefs while they dance.

The traditional art of taekwondo today clearly provides more than proficiency in combat skills; it instills a sense of self-worth and well being. Hope in life is revived inasmuch as seeds of passion are planted from the day the student first begins training and is nurtured through years of vigorous, enthusiastic practice. By remaining steadfast in our search for excellence, we become sufficiently confident in our abilities to convey the spirit through artful expression and living the martial way.

Yet, in spite of artistic articulation, diverse influences projected by rival nations, master instructors convinced of the authenticity of their individual styles, and staggering cultural whirlwinds, taekwondo claims a legacy all its own. This unique heritage can be traced back to an era when scholar-warriors roamed the countryside defending against the onslaughts of imperialistic forces bent on regional domination. Consequently, as we shall see, their triumphs are in no small part responsible for the growth and permanence of traditional taekwondo and the nation we know today as Korea.

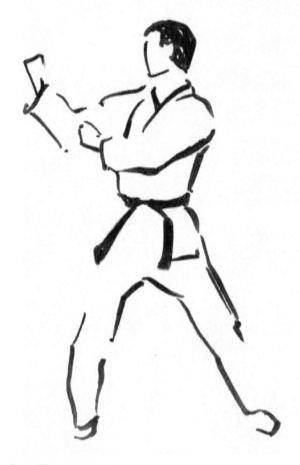

Part Two

An Honorable
History

The Birth of a Nation:
The Ancient Myth of Tangoon

Long ago, before the first kick was thrown, before the blocks and strikes of taekwondo were canonized, there existed a land, rich in greenery with mountains masked in swirling mists that rushed to meet the sky. It was a time when animals were thought to speak and heaven and earth were one. Legend tells us that it was here in these Eastern lands, during the year 2333 B.C., that the divine being Hwanin commanded his son Hwanung to descend from heaven and inhabit the pinnacle of Mount Baekdoo, a sacred place, with express instructions to carve a new country from the primordial terrain. Hwanung, who personified the virtues of honor, courage, and trust, brought with him the Wind-General, the Rain-Governor, and the Cloud-Teacher, along with three thousand lesser spirits to help support his efforts. Together they established Shinshi, the mythical Divine City.

Not far from Shinshi, in a small cave engraved in the rock, dwelt a lumbering bear and a fierce tiger who in their own way desired to become human. Upon overhearing the prayers of the bear and tiger, Hwanung offered to grant their wish under the condition that they remain secluded in the cave for a period of one hundred days, eating nothing but the twenty garlic cloves and artemisia provided. Because of the tiger's innate restlessness, after twenty days he was unable to meet this demand. The bear, on the other hand, whose patience prevailed, exited the cave as a beautiful maiden and was given the name Ungyo, or "the girl incarnated from a bear." Hwanung was so taken with Ungyo's magnificence that he asked her to become his bride. Miraculously, following

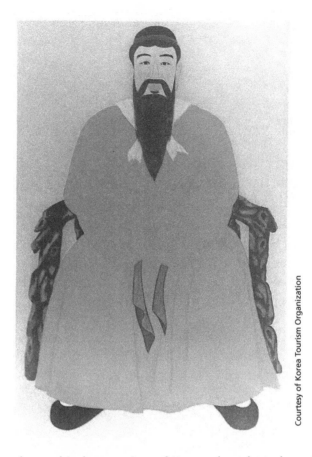

Courtesy of Korea Tourism Organization

Tangoon, the mythical progenitor of Korea, thought to have lived in 2333 B.C.

the transmission of Hwanung's breath of life, she gave birth to a son, naming him Tangoon or "Lord of the Birch Trees." Raised by the ancients, Tangoon went on to help civilize the uncultivated clans by teaching them farming, architecture, and various social graces.[19]

After uniting the six northern tribes, Tangoon, considered the progenitor of modern-day Korea, established the nation of Ko-Chosun, the "Land of the Morning Calm." More importantly, the mythical founder, purported to have ruled until 1122 B.C., is credited with the origination of a traditional, national philosophy through his advocacy of hongik-ingan, the benefits of universal humanism through harmony, and jaese-ihwa, the rationalization of human living.[20] These concepts, based on Confucian thought, codify the Korean sense of duty to the state, family, and forebears, and constitute the foundation of a social framework that has blossomed into the uniquely Korean culture that exists today. Furthermore, the ancients needed to reconcile the ruthlessness of the elements, natural phenomenon, and a highly restrictive lifestyle by clinging to a belief in heaven's god, or impeccable virtuousness that later became defined as seon. Subsequently, these doctrines contributed much to the *do*, or *The Way* of taekwondo, as well as shaping the overall character of traditional and contemporary Korean ethics.

The Three Kingdoms Period: Battlegrounds of Honor

Ancient legends aside, the martial tradition of taekwondo can be traced back to a primitive era in Korean history categorized as the Three Kingdoms Period. Koguryo, the largest of the three, is alleged to have been founded in 37 B.C. along the Yalu River and encompassed an area with landholdings reaching far up into what is now North Korea and Manchuria. A society given to a militaristic worldview, ancient Chinese records describe the Koguryoan people as fond of raiding, quick-tempered, extremely violent, yet courageous. As a result of daily military exercises, it is said that their walking stride was as fast as running.

Due to its close proximity to the vastness of China, the kingdom was in constant conflict with its imperialistic neighbor. Early on, Koguryo forces were intent on the expulsion of the Chinese command posts at Nang-nang, setting the stage for countless, future battles. A reflection of the kingdom's aggressive nature can be seen in the actions of Ulchi Mundok, a cunning military commander who, in A.D. 612, waged war against the recently unified Chinese Sui dynasty. Using deception as a tool, he entered

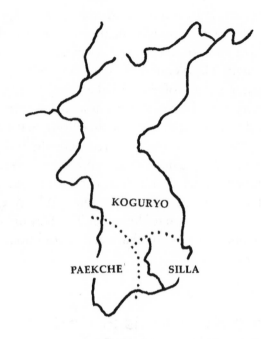

the enemy camp in mock surrender while gauging his adversary's preparedness for battle. Believing his intentions sincere, the Chinese released him only to see their army of over one million ultimately vanquished at his hands.

In answer to a continual fear of invasion, the ruling aristocracy established a warrior corps that came to be known as the *Sunbae*. Literally translated as "wise senior," Sunbae philosophy underscored a deep belief in the gods who created the universe coupled with a strong will to defend the country against all odds. These philosopher/warriors, selected from all rungs of society, dressed in black velvet robes and were required to shave their heads. The Sunbae hierarchal structure was such that anyone given high aptitude and an ambitious character could obtain superior rank. Using this select group of soldiers as a blueprint for its own design, the tiny kingdom of Silla would later create a similar warrior corps whose legendary triumphs would echo down the halls of Korean martial arts for generations to come.

Chinese fighting systems utilized against Koguryo warriors very likely influenced modern taekwondo with the introduction of circular kicking and striking skills. Most sources agree that *taekkyon*, the indigenous Korean martial discipline featuring many of these circular kicking techniques, contributed greatly to the formulation of taekwondo during its formative years. Aside from these practical combat applications, cultural remnants of Koguryo martial arts exist in the form of murals painted on the ceiling of Muyong-chong, a royal tomb located in southern Manchuria built between A.D. 3 and A.D. 427. Shown there are two men engaged in what appears to be a form of sparring that faintly resembles the taekwondo techniques of today.

Paekche, the second largest of the three kingdoms, was established in 18 B.C. It is purported to have developed from a single tribe and was located in the southwest portion of the Korean peninsula. Where historians label Koguryo as characteristically austere and authoritarian, Paekche bears the reputation for being opportunistic and effete. Its people studied archery, horseback riding, and enjoyed a highly developed culture superior at the time to both Koguryo and Silla. As early as the fifth century, in what would later evolve into an alliance of convenience, state scholars were sent across the sea to Japan for the purpose of transmitting the Chinese classics to Japanese citizens.

In the year A.D. 400, the Paekche leadership sought to maximize its relationship with Japan by combining forces in an effort to dominate the entire territory south of Koguryo. To the east lay the tiny kingdom of Silla, a nation-state that would eventually exert the greatest influence, not only on the traditional martial art of taekwondo but on the Korean consciousness as a whole. In a strategic move intended to repulse the impending invasion that threatened Sillian sovereignty, King Naemul requested reinforcements from his counterpart in Koguryo. King Gwanggaeto responded by sending an estimated contingent of 50,000 troops. Along with their strength in numbers, these warriors brought with them knowledge of *kwonbop*, an advanced system of empty-hand fighting skills unique to the region. These techniques undoubtedly supplemented the combat skills of *subyeokta*, a native martial art described in the *Haedong-ungi*, a historical record of the time, as a method of self-defense utilizing arms, legs, and hands as swords. The combined effect of these disciplines, too, would influence the future development of taekwondo. Successful in repelling the armies united under the banners of Paekche and Japan, Silla found itself in the untenable position of being internally imposed upon by its Koguryoan allies. In a convoluted turn of events that confirms the often fickle nature of history and following many years of conflict, Silla surprisingly forged an alliance with its recent adversary, Paekche, in A.D. 433, eventually ridding itself of Koguryo's troublesome incursion into its political affairs.

But of all three kingdoms, diminutive Silla, the most ancient, born in 57 B.C. and located in the southeast corner of the peninsula, was destined to leave the brightest hue on the canvas of Korea's golden past. Originally a confederation of the six Chin-han clans, the tiny kingdom managed to retain many of its ritual traditions, characteristics, and customs where other cultures had failed. It became a refuge of sorts for those preferring a conservative way of life rather than existing in a society overshadowed by authoritarian rule. Demonstrating a desire for practicality, the nation's iron resources were forged into religious icons, farming implements, kitchenware, temple bells, and jewelry, rather than being used exclusively for military purposes. It should come as no surprise then that Kyongju, its capital, was home to over one million inhabitants—a population almost five times that of today's.

With a social fabric woven with strong Confucian and Buddhist fibers, the Sillian leadership evolved by reorganizing the government, consolidating its citizenry, and creating institutions commensurate with the times. By way of example, during the reign of King Pophung, the "true-bone" system was established. Similar to an aristocratic scheme of castes, a person's hereditary bloodline determined the type of home he could dwell in, the clothing he could wear, the food he was permitted to eat, even the method of transportation that carried him from place to place.

At the pinnacle stood royalty, followed by the nobility, with the peasantry finishing last in rank. Kings and queens were considered sacred-bones, or *seonggol*, while their offspring were designated *jingol*, or true-bones. This inequitable social order would contribute to the hierarchal structure fostered by the Hwarang—an elite warrior corps similar to Paekche's Sunbae, which would ultimately unite the warring Three Kingdoms and inspire the martial art of taekwondo in centuries to come.

The Way of the Flowering Manhood: Hwarang-do

Nestled in the emerald folds of Nam-san Mountain, overlooking the majestic Kyongju Plain, sits Tong-Il Jeon Shrine, a memorial to the unification of the Three Kingdoms and to the Hwarang—the elite group of illustrious warriors directly responsible for bringing the Korean peninsula under common rule for the first time in recorded history.

While visiting this memorial, I passed meditation gardens wetted by serene pools teeming with aquatic plants of all varieties.

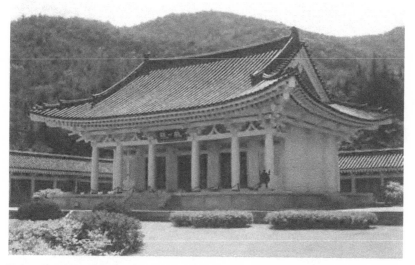

Tong-Il Jeon Shrine, located in Kyongju, South Korea, memorializes venerable warriors and royalty of the Silla kingdom.

Then I climbed countless steps in order to reach stately structures housing dynamic oil paintings of military training and legendary battles; attached beneath each frame is a brass plaque etched with words describing the action. Protected from the elements by the gracefully scalloped roofs so prevalent in Asian culture, it quickly became apparent that these pieces of art depict a timeline steeped in honor and bravery. Through the brushstrokes of a skillful artist, courageous deeds and acts of chivalry carried out by a select force of combatants were painstakingly captured on canvas for the entire world to see.

At the core of this sacred compound stands a central structure guarded by two bipedal turtles mounted on granite pedestals. Enshrined within hang massive portraits of King Muyeol, King Munmu, and General Kim Yu Shin, military commander, architect of unification, and disciple of Hwarang-do—*The Way of the Flowering Manhood*. The man General Kim became, as well as others like him, was forged on the anvil of this unique and demanding discipline. Who were these selfless patriots who served their king

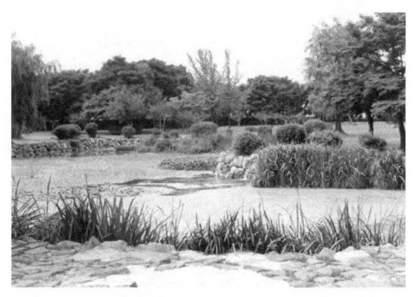

Meditation gardens add to the grandeur of Tong-Il Jeon Shrine.

unconditionally? What secret instruction did they receive? And how did they differ from the rank and file troops of their era?

Founded by King Jin Heung in A.D. 37, the Hwarang represented a fraternity of Silla's noble elite composed of intelligent young men drawn from prestigious families. Compared with military cadets of our time, the Hwarang are arguably seen by some as the forerunners of the samurai. Their numbers were renowned for exhibiting extraordinary martial valor when acting as vanguards on the field of battle. Aside from their knowledge of *kwonbop* and *subak*, two native martial arts of the day, the youthful warriors of the Hwarang were distinguished from other combat troops by virtue of their unique holistic schooling in archery, dance, poetry, music, equestrian skills, and martial arts and were supported by a deep belief in the Eastern philosophical paradigms of Confucianism, Buddhism, and Taoism. Patterned after the Sunbae of Koguryo, the Hwarang evolved from six elementary garrisons established by the Sillian leadership. These defensive contingents referred to as *chong* were distributed throughout the six provinces and commanded by superiors of "true-bone" status. With experienced officers designated as

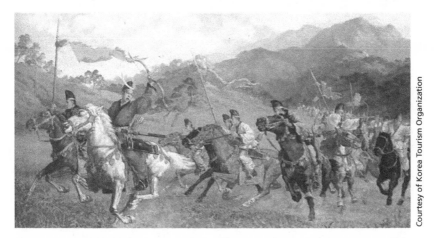

Courtesy of Korea Tourism Organization

Warriors of the Hwarang practiced martial arts and acted in accordance with the philosophical paradigms of Confucianism, Buddhism, and Taoism.

kukson, or national seniors supervising smaller units consisting of eight troops, members of the Hwarang were often flagged for esteemed military command and vital government positions. Hwarang youth were well prepared for these high stations since they lived under a strict code of honor handed down by the Buddhist monk, Wonkwang Popsa, a pivotal figure in the ethical development of modern taekwondo. These basic, moral principles included loyalty to the king, filial piety, and restraint against the misuse of force in battle. When not engaged in combat, Hwarang warriors were known to make pilgrimages ritualizing the prosperity of their nation through song and dance, provide support to those experiencing difficult times, make repairs to roads and castles, and undertake rigorous martial arts training in the high mountains and deep valleys of the region.

Stirrings of Buddhist Thought in Taekwondo: Wonkwang, Kwisan, and Chuhang

Considering the sophistication of the order, Hwarang-do provided fertile ground for the growth of future kings, generals, and statesmen destined to guide the kingdom from relative obscurity to its legendary position as an influential regional power. Several great examples of acquired strength through the search for spiritual enrichment, intense training, and bone-rank status are the deeds and actions of Kwisan, Chuhang, the boy-warrior Kwanch'ang, and General Kim Yu Shin, whose exploits ring clear in the annuls of Korean history. It is almost impossible to accurately portray the impassioned narratives and exploits that took place in the late seventh century between these luminaries, particularly Wonkwang Popsa and two inquisitive Hwarang warriors, mostly due to the fragmentary manner in which the overall history of the Korean martial arts have been documented. Yet if we were to journey back in time to the age of the Hwarang, perhaps the transmission of this ancient wisdom, at least as I see it, would have taken place something like this:

A full moon shone against an ebony sky, its light falling diagonally through the slender branches of the birch trees that rocked gently in the autumn breeze. Although it was well after midnight, Kwisan was restless, tossing and turning on the pine needles he and his loyal comrade had gathered to make their beds. Chuhang slept peacefully across the clearing, warmed by the receding embers of the fire from the night before. It had been a long, arduous journey and the two companions took delight in knowing that their destination drew near.

For some time now this pair of young warriors had shared a concern stemming from the wanton bloodshed they observed almost daily, perpetrated by undisciplined troops on the field of battle. Realizing that their common adversaries fought to preserve the national honor and dignity of their respective kingdoms just as they did, it seemed overly cruel to indiscriminately take life so brutally when not directly threatened.

But the benevolent thoughts and complex concerns of these men were unique in the history of Asian warfare since they were no ordinary soldiers. Instead of being kin to the folk that composed the rank and file army defending the tiny kingdom of Silla to which they belonged, Kwisan and Chuhang were warriors of the Hwarang. With minds unsullied by cynicism they reasoned: Should not this respect for life be universal regardless of borders? They were confident that the answers to this question and others concerning purification of the mind would be made apparent to them in the days ahead.

After rising and consuming the morning meal, they mounted their steeds that till now stood grazing in the grassy field beyond. Both young men felt optimistic about their upcoming audience with the Buddhist monk,

Wonkwang Popsa. Acknowledged far and wide for his compassion and wisdom, the elderly sage, now fifty-nine years of age, was currently residing at Hwangnyong Temple and even now was extolling the virtues of the Buddhist faith at the Assembly of One Hundred Seats.

Kwison and Chuhang traveled through that entire day and into the night uninterrupted, feeling their anticipation rise with each hoof beat. Exhausted after gingerly picking their way through brambles and hoping their horses would not stumble on the narrow, rock strewn path that precipitously wound its way down the mountain toward the vast expanse of the Kyongju Plain, the young warriors at last caught their first glimpse of the temple walls silhouetted by the rising sun. Passing monks foraging for the few sticks of firewood so scarce in that environment, the pair passed through the ornate portal of the spiritual compound. Once dismounted, their road-weary horses were stabled.

Kwisan and Chuhang were silently led by a group of weathered monks toward a central temple where a congregation from throughout the kingdom had assembled to witness the ministrations of Wonkwang. Upon entering the vast hall, it was difficult to see, given the contrast between the dimly lit interior and the brightening sky outside. Clouds of incense, so intense that they were intoxicating, suffused the air. Those participating in the morning's first meditation practice were dispersing to enjoy a meager breakfast. Kwisan and Chuhang passed through the throng and humbly approached the master's door. Beckoned to enter, they raised their robes in the Confucian custom of greeting. Kneeling before the sacred master who was leaning on a tall staff and adorned in a gray undergarment covered by a scarlet robe, Kwisan respectfully intoned: "We are ignorant and devoid of knowledge. Please convey to us principles which will serve to instruct us for all the days of our lives." The great master Wonkwang replied there are ten injunctions in the Bodhisattva ordination. "But, since you are subjects and sons," he continued, "I fear you cannot practice them all. Here, however, are five directives for laymen. The first is to serve your King with loyalty. Second, tend your parents with filial piety. Next, treat your friends with consideration and sincerity. Fourth, do not retreat in the face of battle. And, finally, be discriminating concerning the taking of life. Though you may have need, do not kill often. These," the kind monk concluded, "are the good rules for laymen." Rising in unison, the two Hwarang bowed in supplication and left the chamber feeling gifted with a shared knowledge that would ultimately travel down the centuries to shape the very fabric of Korean and tae-kwondo ethical principles.

Documented in the *Samguk Yusa* (*Lives of Eminent Korean Monks*),[21] the *Sesok Ogye* or "The Five Codes of Human Conduct" advocated by Wonkwang, contained a mixture of Buddhist and Confucian doctrine and quickly became the *Warrior Oath of the Hwarang* after being transmitted to Kwisan and Chuhang in A.D. 613.[22] These ancient moral directives eventually evolved into what is widely recognized today as the *Student Creed of Taekwondo*. As cultures merged, however, it was expanded to instill trust between teachers and students, fidelity in marriage, respect for elders, and perseverance in deeds and actions. We wonder who in the distant past could have predicted that the ethical curiosity exhibited by two young Sillian warriors would result in the prominent posting of these principles in dojangs, or training halls, around the globe with the intention of promoting honorable behavior in martial artists of all ages and backgrounds.

As it reads today, these moral precepts include:

STUDENT CREED OF TAEKWONDO
1. Be loyal to your country.
2. Be loving and show fidelity to your parents.
3. Be loving between husband and wife.
4. Be cooperative between brothers and sisters.
5. Be faithful to your friends.
6. Be respectful to your elders.
7. Establish trust between teacher and student.
8. Use good judgment before harming any living thing.
9. Never retreat in battle.
10. Always finish what you start.

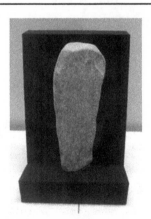

A stone tablet thought to have been inscribed by Kwisan and Chuhang, describing the basic ideology of Hwarang-do.

As a testament to the timelessness surrounding the ten noble principles that comprise the cornerstone of the Korean martial arts, many training halls routinely call for their recitation at the close of a practice session. Moreover, they are directly related to the tenets dictated by the *Sesok Ogye* and now more than ever remain a dynamic blueprint for ethical conduct. Not to be construed as a neighborly set of values or the casual lines of some benevolent verse, this creed represents a direct link to the past and a reflection of the true essence surrounding the practice of traditional taekwondo.

The Legend of Kwan-ch'ang, The Boy-Warrior

Yet another example of the leadership and valor exhibited under the teachings of Hwarang-do was that set by Kwan-ch'ang, who at age 16 was already an assistant general under his father, General P'umil. Adding credence to the ninth directive of the *Student Creed of Taekwondo*—never retreat in battle—the actions of the boy-warrior continue to inspire many adherents to Korean culture to this day. Following a number of setbacks during an important battle with Paekche in A.D. 660, Kwan-ch'ang's father requested that he rally his forces and rouse the troops of the other generals. In the midst of battle, the boy warrior galloped into the enemy camp leaving a trail of vanquished adversaries in his wake. Kwan-ch'ang was taken captive and brought before General Ge-Baek, commanding officer of the Paekche forces. Astonished by both the courage and youthfulness of the prisoner, the General exclaimed, "This is only a boy! Alas for us if we cannot match such courage. If these are the exploits of a boy, what must we expect from their men?" At this point, realizing the valor in the deed, the commander ordered the young man to be allowed safe passage and return to his camp unharmed. But no sooner had Kwan-ch'ang been released than he reentered the fray, spearing many opponents along the way. After being recaptured, as punishment, he was this time decapitated and his head sent back to the Sillian troops tied to his horse's saddle. Rather than being viewed as a tragedy, however, Kwan-ch'ang's father lifted the head from the saddle with the pronouncement, "My son's honor lives! I have no regret that he gave his life for his king." The Sillian army deeply moved and inspired by such virtuous action went on that day to obtain a decisive victory over the Paekche forces.

General Kim Yu Shin: Architect of Unification

Born in A.D. 595, it is said that Kim Yu Shin was the great-grand-child of King Kuhae, assuring him "true-bone" status in accordance with the hierarchal structure of Sillian culture. An avid disciple of Hwarang-do, by the age of fifteen he acquired great skill as a swordsman advancing to the rank of kukson in his eighteenth year. By age thirty-four, he was given total command of the Sillian armed forces.

While still a young man, Kim Yu Shin observed the aggressive tendencies of Koguryo and Paekche, resolving early on to terminate their predatory intentions. Retiring to a stone grotto deep within the Diamond Mountains, the Hwarang warrior fasted and purified his spirit through meditation. In patriotic fervor, he swore an oath to heaven saying: "The unprincipled enemies harass our lands like wolves and tigers, and peace has departed from the earth. I am but one insignificant subject, lacking the strength or skill but determined to remove these misfortunes and disorders. If only heaven could be moved to send me some assistance."[23]

After he remained in solitude for four days, legend has it that an elderly sage attired in coarse garments approached him. Revering his resolve and sincere desire to unite the Three Kingdoms, the old man provided Kim with secret principles and training involving the martial arts. His teachings, however, were tempered with cautionary advice urging against the misuse of fighting skills which would surely lead to disaster. Satisfied that his task was complete, the stranger turned and departed the stone grotto. Wishing to express his gratitude, Yu Shin pursued his benefactor only to discover a cloud of light pervading the mountaintop where he had once stood.

But perhaps the most colorful legend involving General Kim Yu Shin is that describing his ingenuity in battle. Transforming what could potentially have been a disaster of immense proportions into a stunning defeat, this tale demonstrates the results of a shrewd mind coupled with the indomitable will inherent in Korean culture:

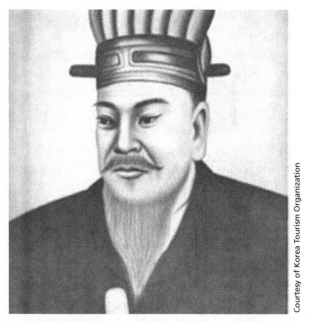

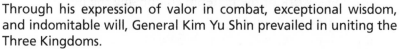

Through his expression of valor in combat, exceptional wisdom, and indomitable will, General Kim Yu Shin prevailed in uniting the Three Kingdoms.

The blackened clouds had gathered quickly, exploding in an electric fury beyond all memory. Thunderous reports from heaven were accompanied by a drenching rain that pelted ceaselessly down, causing the tunics of the exhausted warriors to become saturated, adding to the weight of their already burdensome armor. The campfires that had provided warmth and light were long ago extinguished by the downpour.

Shortly before the ungodly deluge began, an uncanny sight filled the night sky. A star had fallen to the earth, thrust from its rightful place in the universe by a vengeful deity intent on the destruction of those with the unsanctioned audacity to wage war. Viewed instantly by the bedraggled and superstitious combatants as an omen of defeat, the seasoned legion—men who had fought valiantly through endless battles—lost its senses, cowered, and ran about in circles.

General Kim Yu Shin shook his head from side to side and quietly swore beneath his breath. He had been ordered by the king to subdue a rebel force of extraordinary strength that threatened the capital. Before the fiery visitor from above made its appearance, his army had dominated the battlefield. Now, control of his men was rapidly evaporating, along with the impact of each raindrop. What creative method could he employ to regain the initiative and rally his troops?

Casting about in the ensuing mayhem, he spied his command tent and the tightly-stretched fabric that protected its interior from the elements; an idea began to take hold in his head. An accomplished swordsman of wide renown, he drew his blade from the scabbard making quick work of the material comprising the north side of the shelter. Within seconds several pieces of the rough fabric lay on the wet ground before him. Connecting tree branches to the corners of one particularly large section, he constructed a box-shaped kite of enormous proportions. Summoning the aid of his lieutenants, he gathered the remaining sections into a single, large ball and ordered that it be submerged for some minutes in a barrel containing fuel for the torches. Satisfied with the results of his work, he carefully connected the curious object to the kite's tail.

Clandestinely dragging the assembled contraption up a steep hill with his soldiers assisting, General Kim hefted the kite aloft, but not before igniting the fuel-drenched ball dangling from its end. Running vigorously against the wind, the hemp line rapidly uncoiled as the luminous object swiftly rose skyward. To the watchful eyes of those on the field of battle, the fallen star—that vivid portent of disaster—had miraculously ascended once again, retrieved by the gods, seemingly as a symbol of absolution.

Heartened by the brilliant fireball clearly thought to be a sign from above, a roar of triumph emanated from the throats of thousands of Kim's troops, provoking fear and confusion in the enemy camp. With sword held high, lightning reflecting off its carefully-tooled surface, General Kim astride his steed seized the moment, driving his men forward on the road to honor.

Due to the resourcefulness of its supreme commander in using a supposed weapon triggered by a divine source, a decisive victory was won for the tiny kingdom of Silla. Using his kite as a model, a system of aerial signals was devised by General Kim that would later evolve into a method of communication between troops separated by great distances.

Through his expression of valor in combat, exceptional wisdom, and indomitable will, General Kim prevailed in uniting the Three Kingdoms while earning great merit and fame. With the aid of Chinese forces and skillful diplomacy, Silla ultimately succeeded in the conquest of Paekche in A.D. 663, and finally, Koguryo in A.D. 668. So what began as a loose confederation of bickering tribes, now answered to a single monarch under the banner of United Silla.

Regarded as the driving force in the unification of the Korean peninsula, Kim Yu Shin lived to the age of seventy-eight. He was handsomely rewarded for his accomplishments by being given extensive land holdings accompanied by the undying respect of a nation. Upon his death in A.D. 673, he was laid to rest at the foot of Songhwa Mountain in Kyongju in a tomb appropriately fit for a king.

In the Footsteps of Hwarang-do: The Influence of Ancient Warriors

Today, practitioners of taekwondo and Korean society at large look to illustrious members of the Hwarang, such as Kim Yu Shin and others like him, for inspiration when adversity strikes. Unlike pugilistic pursuits that stress victory in the ring at all costs, traditional taekwondo rests on a foundation of virtuous action. Viewed through the lens of history, the taekwondoist draws strength from the supreme examples set by the disciples of Hwarang-do in coping with the struggles life presents as well as the joys it offers, through the experience of elevated learning and martial discipline. While kicks, blocks, and strikes make up the physical component of taekwondo, the moral aspect of this unique Korean martial art revolves around many of the virtues practiced by the Hwarang.

But the growth of the Korean martial arts that would one day evolve into the modern discipline of taekwondo did not end with the unification of Koguryo, Paekche, and Silla, nor with the emergence of the Koryo (A.D. 918-1392) and Chosun (Yi) (A.D. 1392-1910) dynasties. Rather, the ways of unarmed combat would ride up and down on the shifting tides of Korean culture, through periods necessitating a strong defensive posture coupled with centuries of neglect at the hands of those seeing the practical application of the martial arts as contradictory to the philosophical principles of the times. As fate would have it, the Korean people would pay dearly for these extended lapses in martial arts training particularly during the Chosun Dynasty. But for now, that time had not yet come and a period of peace and prosperity was to reign over the Korean peninsula both for the Hwarang and for the subjects of United Silla in general.

The Koryo and Chosun Dynasties

The 475 years following the United Silla era represented a time of growth and reorganization. Thirty-seven kings ruled over wondrous advances that became the trademark of the Koryo Dynasty. In A.D. 1234, moveable metal type was invented, preceding Guttenberg by 200 years. Developed by native artisans, Koryo celadon, noted for its colorful green and blue glaze, can be found in museums around the world and continues to capture the attention of collectors to this day. Korean Buddhism embraced a martial component during this period in the form of the Subdue Demon Corps who are credited with holding off the Jurchen invaders. Fighting monks bearing martial arts skills were not uncommon.

As a religious paradigm, however, Buddhism began to wane in favor of the more practical teachings of Confucius.

The Chosun Dynasty, last of the great dynastic successions, gave rise to many noted leaders and military tacticians. During the decline of the Koryo Dynasty, the virtuous effects of Buddhism had spun out of control, poisoning the upper echelons of government. Leaders were required to become Buddhist monks as a prerequisite to kingship. As a backlash to the abuses of the Buddhist priesthood, Confucianism became the dominant philosophy allowing civilians, rather than the clergy, to fill the halls of power. Appallingly, the practice of native martial arts faded into the background during the Chosun Dynasty, in no small part due to the introduction of gunpowder and other technological advances on the battlefield.

The brightest jewel in the crown of cultural achievement during this era was set by King Sejong, who reigned from A.D. 1418-1450. One of the most revered leaders in Korean history, King Sejong was responsible for the invention of *hangul*, the unique Korean alphabet consisting of 24 letters and lauded by linguists for its accuracy in phonetically representing the sounds of native words. Known as the "Leonardo da Vinci" of the region for his talents and innovation, King Sejong was also involved in the development of timepieces, rain gauges, and a 365-volume medical encyclopedia.

Until the latter part of the eighteenth century the Chosun people, with their nation being dubbed "The Hermit Kingdom," were largely unaware of the comings and goings of the Western world. This narrow global view was about to be inextricably altered with the introduction of Catholicism, rumors of technological advances heralded by traveling envoys, new bloodlines introduced by ship-wrecked sailors, and the political manipulations of the major world powers, all of whom were equally guilty in turning a deaf ear to the cries of a nation that was about to suffer humiliation at the hands of Japanese colonialism.

In the years that ensued, from A.D. 1910 to 1945, the Japanese attempted, by force, to eradicate all vestiges of Korean society.

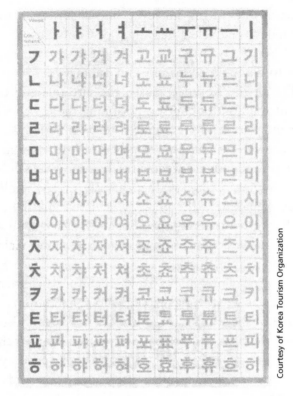

Created by King Sejong in 1443, hangul permitted the average citizen to access classical literature.

Politics trumped compassion in a battle of cultures. It would ultimately take over three decades and a world war to extricate the Korean people from the clutches of imperialism.

The Politics of Taekwondo Today

Just as in Korean history, everywhere we turn today we see the effects of politics. Politics have a profound influence on the future of world events including the way we work, the food we eat, and the air we breathe. In fact, even traditional taekwondo is not immune to the long shadow cast by politics. After becoming familiar with the development of the Korean martial arts, this should come as no surprise. Historical evidence demonstrates that following the period of United Silla, King Uijong of the Koryo Dynasty used subak, an early form of taekwondo, as a yardstick in measuring the competency of his military commanders. And once anything is coupled to government it begins to resonate with political overtones. But the use of politics as a tool is not unique to national governments. In fact, politics can manifest its power between disparate organizations, groups, or individuals. This becomes abundantly clear when we consider the true definition of politics which can be construed as *who gets what, when, and how*.[24]

Clearly, traditional taekwondo is replete with an enhanced set of moral principles as typified by the Five Tenets and the Student Creed of Taekwondo. As sincere practitioners, many of us would like to think that these virtues have the ability to elevate our art above the political fray. Yet this is simply not the case. Nor is it entirely bad. Just as fire—a natural force—is indifferent to good and evil, political intent in and of itself is blind to inequity. It is what humanity makes of these things that ultimately determine their perspective and value. At best, political discourse can provide a resolution for debate. At worst, it can usher in despotism and suffering.

Over the course of time, taekwondo has been tossed on a sea of political manipulation, riding the crest of a wave one moment only to be swallowed by a deep trough the next. For example, the turbulent years that spanned the first half of the twentieth century prior to 1945 were rudely influenced by the Japanese Occupation of Korea and found many native martial artists whose lives were in jeopardy, by virtue of their art, emigrating to Japan or China where they were assigned work, or worse, conscripted to serve the very military machine that was actively crushing their homeland. Here in these foreign lands Korean masters were oddly not only permitted to practice the martial arts forbidden by imperial rule back home, but earned advancement and teaching credentials as well. Pivotal figures such as General Choi Hong Hi, Won

Kuk Lee, and Hwang Kee were beneficiaries of this dubious political aberration. Borrowing from a variety of provincial styles, these pioneers and others like them would later return to Korea, then under a different sort of domination, albeit more benign, to launch or create martial arts and enduring organizations of their own with a distinctly Korean flavor yet colored by cultural impressions and methods accumulated abroad.[25]

Later, in 1955, politics again would sculpt the future of taekwondo at a conference considering unification of the various kwans or schools existing at the time. Now-famous institutes such as the Moo Duk Kwan (Institute of Martial Virtue), Chung Do Kwan (Institute of the Blue Waves), and Chang Moo Kwan (Martial Spirit Training Institute) were strongly urged by the Korean government to renounce the accepted term tangsoodo (way of the China hand) in favor of the newly-coined phrase taekwondo (foot, hand, way) in perhaps a subconscious effort to reclaim a national identity seriously injured by a brutal interloper. Today, most historians agree that it was General Choi Hong Hi who, on April 11, 1955, created the name taekwondo based on its close association with the indigenous Korean kicking art taekkyon rather than support an imprimatur gleaned from a foreign nation. Several of the masters in attendance at this critical meeting were comfortable with their present method of teaching and found the concept of merging styles objectionable. Great hurdles needed to be overcome before any decision could be made. Once an agreement was reached, the specter of politics again played an important role in the maturation process of taekwondo when General Choi was urged to obtain permission from then-President Syngman Rhee to use the new name. Following much debate, consent was finally granted.

Today, as in times past, political debate continues to surround taekwondo. Organizations, such as the IOC and the WTF, now under the direction of Dr. Chung Won Choue, have done much to promote taekwondo as an Olympic sport yet are often looked upon as diluting the traditional essence of the art. By the same token, the ITF—perceived somewhat as the champion

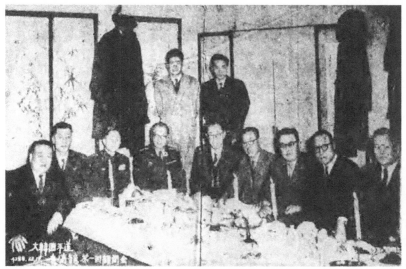

Courtesy of Tae Kwon Do Times

The April 11, 1955 meeting where the art of taekwondo was named. General Choi Hong Hi is seated third from left.

of traditional taekwondo and brainchild of General Choi Hong Hi—has been seeking Olympic participation for years while maintaining an emphasis on classical self-defense. Then there exist institutions similar to the USTA, presided over by Grandmaster Richard Chun that actively address both the martial art *and* martial sport of taekwondo.

Clearly, politics have played a major role in molding the current model of taekwondo as we know it today. In retrospect, if the political leadership of the Chosun Dynasty had not been forced by military necessity to resurrect its native martial arts radically overshadowed by the rise of Confucianism, the embryonic style of taekwondo practiced during that period may not have survived at all. Likewise, without the differing views and ultimate agreement arrived at by the kwan (institute) masters of the 1940s and 50s, the Korean martial arts may have limped along as a splintered group of fighting styles lacking any central identity. And, finally, if the WTF had not risen to the Olympic gold standard created by the international sports community, thus catapulting taekwondo to world prominence, the art may have remained simply a provincial set of fighting skills rather than the most popular martial discipline in the world today.[26]

Nevertheless, the political tradition of taekwondo works both ways. Often, in order to gain an advantage in one area we must acquiesce in another, personifying the true essence of politics. Let us hope that the contrasting views of conflicting organizations and individuals will not follow the present tenuous path of world politics, but will be evaluated in a constructive manner permitting taekwondo to continue its evolution as a modern world sport and traditional martial art complete with a rich set of honorable principles by which to live.

Traditional Taekwondo in the 21st Century

The dawning of the twenty-first century has seen much in the way of conflict both on a global and personal level. More than ever, cultural differences coupled with opposing world views appear to have spiraled out of control. The integrity of our most sacred institutions has been brought into question with internal corruption tearing at the roots of government, big business, and even religion. More than ever we find ourselves turning inside for answers. For decades traditional taekwondo has been the perfect medium for cultivating inner strength, extraordinary endurance, and an effective arsenal of defensive skills. Motives for training in the martial arts today range anywhere from gaining proficiency in self-defense and physical fitness to propagating discipline and concentration. While sport and all its trappings can provide an outlet for aggression and create social bonds by way of teambuilding, it is by definition restricted to a set time and place. While organized religion attempts to satisfy an innate desire for spiritual enlightenment, it does nothing to address the physical needs of the individual. Martial arts, on the other hand, if offered in a traditional manner, represent a way of life and a vehicle for self-enrichment through diligent training. Invariably, we will ask how a pursuit so resonant with aggressive overtones can benefit humanity. The solution to this paradox can be found in the realization that the more frequently students train and become proficient in the martial arts, the more they will discover that they have less to defend against. Confidence begins to replace fear. Defensive skills become internalized, resulting in the ability to walk life's path appreciating its simple pleasures rather than being blinded by its daily perils. Now, more than ever, these benefits reflect the true worth of traditional taekwondo training.

With roots dating back to antiquity, the robust philosophical foundation that acted as a code of honor for the Hwarang of ancient Silla continues to support traditional taekwondo in the new millennium and remains as valid today as it was in the seventh century when these noble warriors sought wisdom from its precepts. Certainly, Buddhism and, to a lesser degree, Taoism, served as the cornerstones of this philosophy. Nevertheless, it was Confucianism, with its blueprint rooted in ethical behavior, that flourished during the Chosun Dynasty, manifesting itself in grand form on the social fabric of Korea. Even now we can witness the value of this philosophy when applied to today's troubled times. Confucius taught that a single individual can influence world events through the simple projection of a benevolent state of mind. The Korean proverb *su shin je ga chi guk pyong chun fa* supports this notion, once again confirming the vital role Confucianism played in molding the cultural landscape of the Korean nation. Loosely translated, this dictum states, "peace within the individual brings peace within the family; peace in the family brings peace in the community; peace in the community, peace in the country, and peace throughout the world."[27] As improbable a scenario as this may sound there is little doubt that compassion toward fellow human beings goes a long way. Rather than being isolated in a vacuum, correct action ripples across humanity with the same effect as would a pebble when dropped into a serene pool of water. While we are certain to encounter speed bumps of belligerency on our path to fulfillment we must recall that, by and large, a great majority of our fellow human beings desire peace, prosperity, and understanding as much as we do. What better place to initiate the reaffirmation of these principles than within our own mind, body, and spirit, using the ethical doctrines of traditional taekwondo as a roadmap. Still, for me, the quest for enlightenment, however that may be defined, is a fundamental condition of the art. Often the traveler must first become disillusioned in order to find the true path.

Enlightenment through Disillusion

Traditional taekwondo fills a great majority of the requirements I have come to associate with a life based on theocratic thought. Yet as much as I am devoted to my discipline of choice and the virtues it imbues, I recall being faintly disillusioned with taekwondo on several occasions. This is not unusual or uncommon given the cacophony of confusing events that often threaten to rattle the faith of those expressing even the most unshakable convictions.

The first was when I discovered that taekwondo, in spite of popular belief, was not over two thousand years old as alleged even though, as we have seen, it was rooted in that era. This discovery happened years ago when I was teaching a Poomsae & Philosophy Class at a local dojang. Intent on providing my students with concise and accurate information regarding the history of taekwondo, I developed a class plan based on extensive research. Like many of my colleagues who have made a profession of teaching the martial arts, I began reading everything available on the subject to support my syllabus. A great majority of sources, using supposed archeological discoveries as a foundation, clearly stated that taekwondo was practiced during the Three Kingdoms Period (57 B.C.–A.D. 935) right up to the present.[28] Then one day I read a paper published in a scholarly journal that pretty much shattered that misconception. In it, the author presented solid historical evidence destroying the notion that taekwondo, at least as we know it today, existed prior to the

1950s.[29] "How could this be?" I asked in disbelief. Yet the more I investigated, the more I became convinced that this unbiased work was based on legitimate fact.

Then there was the time I visited a dojang in California owned by a world-famous master instructor only to discover that the curriculum taught there varied greatly from the one supported by the school I was currently attending in New York. Not only was the tempo and structure of the class different, but so were the forms and nomenclature of techniques. Visiting schools across the nation was the result of a habit I had developed when traveling on business. In preparation for my journey, I would routinely call ahead to my destination hotel and request the concierge to fax me a copy of the Yellow Pages advertisements for martial arts schools. Looking for common identifiers such as organizational affiliation, I would seek out dojangs teaching a style similar to my own. Since I traveled frequently in those days, I was presented with a wealth of opportunities to attend a variety of locations. All but one seemed to emphasize different aspects of taekwondo with many even offering mixed martial arts with little or no loyalty to one given style. "Something is desperately wrong here! Taekwondo is an absolute art with no room for this much variation," thought I.

But perhaps the most profound disappointment came when I discovered that even poomsae, that most sacred of practices, were not executed in the same manner at every location. Formal patterns, at least to me, were immutable. Most are documented in exhaustive detail. So, how on earth could there exist even the slightest variation in performance? Forms represent the essence of any classical martial art, the method in which taekwondo in particular was catalogued and handed down over what I had by now understood, was decades. Some forms were even borrowed from martial arts with legacies dating back centuries. How then was it possible for any one individual to even imagine corrupting these timeless sequences of defensive wisdom?

In answer to these questions, let me first acknowledge that age coupled with experience promotes wisdom. Yet earned wisdom is not indiscriminate tolerance for error. In other words, the longer students diligently study taekwondo while adhering to the basic principles inherent in the art, such as integrity and perseverance, the more broadminded they become, expanding their world view of the martial arts and life in general. This statement may at first appear somewhat simplistic in nature. Converting a provincial outlook to one that revolves around a charitable approach to change and diversity based on acquired knowledge is a singular accomplishment in any discipline. Still, maintaining an open mind in regard to differences in style does not dismiss the occasional lapse in memory, or worse, intentional distortion of technique as acceptable practice. Armed with this theory, let me briefly revisit my three disillusionments mentioned above.

In regard to the commonly accepted, largely exaggerated history of taekwondo, great military and cultural triumphs were enjoyed by the Korean people during the Silla and Koryo periods. Even so, the Korean nation was historically ravaged by war and civil strife but never more so than since the turn of the twentieth century. Is it any wonder then that a nation struggling to revive a golden past wrapped in honor and innovation should search its collective consciousness for a remedy representing traditional strengths and values by unifying a loosely knit group of martial arts under the banner of taekwondo and benignly expand its history?

Then there exists the question of continuity relative to differing styles. Clearly, just as in the building trade where a nail is a nail and a brick is a brick, contractors regularly vary the use of standard materials according to their method of construction. The same holds true in the martial arts. While maintaining the technical integrity of the various kicks, blocks, and strikes intrinsic to taekwondo, master instructors emphasize and execute these techniques differently. Simply put, there is no hard and fast rule applicable when it comes to teaching drills, forms, and sparring. Business practices contrast from dojang to dojang too, just as does class duration and emphasis on technique. Still, this does not mean that *traditional* taekwondo is not being taught due primarily to a variance in teaching style.

And lastly, while the key poomsae unique to the WTF, ITF, and the Moo Duk Kwan have been exhaustively mapped, their execution ultimately lays at the mercy of those transmitting them. In my second book, *Traditional Taekwondo: Core Techniques, History, and Philosophy*, I clearly state: "Regardless of the mode by which a poomsae or tul is captured for posterity, whether it is of a physical or electronic nature, it is ultimately the responsibility of today's instructors to cherish, preserve, and transmit the classic forms uncorrupted by lack of knowledge or personal style. Only then are practitioners of the future certain to benefit from this effective and traditional form of self-defense education."[30] Naturally, I continue to stand by this declaration, but it is understandable for an instructor to favor certain techniques that he excels in thereby coloring a form in one way or another. This is an example of human nature and does not necessarily infer ignorance or intentional distortion of custom.

Yes, it has taken me years to realize that my initial frustration with certain aspects of the martial arts has led me to a mature enlightenment through the process of disillusion. But, that is *The Way* of traditional taekwondo and the honorable history we share, is it not?

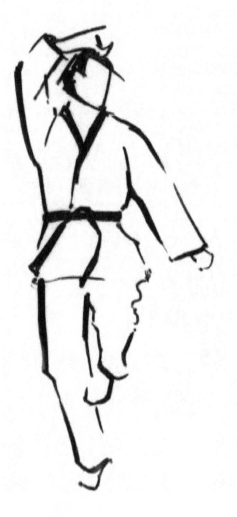

Part Three

Becoming a Steadfast Practitioner

Remaining True to the Art

I am always careful to remind my students that the practice of traditional taekwondo is not easy. I tell them that if it were, everyone would train. And it is not difficult to see why. Movies abound with our favorite stars leaping through the air, chopping, punching, and kicking while making the world right for the meek. Naturally, it is understandable how the average person would identify with these heroes, male and female alike, and wish to emulate them. Yet the true cost of training, both to the practiced and the vanquished, is frequently hidden by the way martial arts are portrayed on television and in the cinema. Not shown are the hours, days, weeks, and years of difficult work the martial artist must put in to develop his technique. Invisible, too, are the deadly consequences of a single well-placed kick or strike. If we were to believe what we see on the screen, we would think that skill sprouts eternal, with little or no effort required to become a true killing machine. Obviously, this is simply not the case. Nor is death and destruction the ultimate goal of the martial artist. In order to become proficient in the traditional martial arts, the practitioner must possess a tireless commitment and undying passion. He must be willing to forego leisure time activities that are often more entertaining. He must also exhibit the capacity to endure sore muscles, aching joints, and an occasional bruise or two. But above all, an abundant supply of patience is essential.

For most of us, the mind has the ability to retain information far more efficiently than our muscles. We must convince our bodies that we are capable of moving in ways that have abandoned many of us since childhood. To observe my adult students, who not long ago were prematurely rooted to the earth due to age, execute jump turning kicks coupled with focused strikes is confirmation enough that taekwondo is a truly liberating force. Children too are challenged, not based on agility or aerobic quality as are their more mature counterparts, but by coordination, balance, and strength. Still, with patience, encouragement, and indomitable will, they excel. Skills of this nature do not come easily. Determination and an unswerving faith in taekwondo are paramount. This devotion is not misplaced even though, admittedly, taekwondo is not the solution to every offensive threat. Yet with thousands of battle-proven techniques at his disposal the taekwondoist should, through patience and practice, cultivate the proper defensive tools for use against almost any threat.

This leads us to the question of cross-training—the practice of actively mixing styles. As a rule of thumb, it is said that a martial artist devoted to a particular discipline should remain faithful to that art for a minimum of seven to eight years before cross-training. Why is this?

First, the martial artists must learn the fundamentals of their art. Without strong basic skills, everything else will falter. This process is generally accomplished during the students' years as a color belt—and then, at black belt, their training truly begins. The path to success in the martial arts unavoidably takes time and if approached with sincerity will provide the practitioner with the tools necessary to continue the journey with confidence—a journey, thankfully, with no foreseeable end.

When considering cross-training, thought should be given to cultural implications and how they relate to a particular martial art. In the past, geography played an influential role on technical development. On another level, so did a nation's history and worldview. Martial arts for many nations, including Korea, historically represented primary instruments of war and were successfully exported to the present as evidenced in taekwondo being used during the Vietnam War.[31]

Nations with a history of repeated invasions and strife had to develop practical martial arts capable of not only defending physically, but emotionally as well. These physical and emotional imprints, for good or ill, often prejudice the underlying philosophy of a given martial art. Subsequently, toggling between differing cultural viewpoints can prove confusing for the martial artist that lacks the maturity to appreciate these distinctions.

Additionally, it is recommended that the practitioner remain focused on a single art due to its technical complexity. Simply put, memorization and proper execution of the countless blocks, strikes, kicks, formal patterns, and defensive strategies that compose traditional taekwondo leave little room for the infiltration of potentially conflicting philosophies and skills. This concept is apparent when stances found in taekwondo are compared to those shared in the martial arts of Japanese and Chinese origin.

For my part, traditional taekwondo is sufficiently complex to keep me busy for a lifetime. With every advanced poomsae, il su sik, or ho sin sool I perform, I appreciate all the more the road that lies before me—the effort that remains to take my practice one step closer to the core of the art. These increments are small, not the dramatic leaps and bounds experienced by the novice. Yet, as the years go by, I eagerly pursue my training, training punctuated with *purpose* and *concentrated martial intent,* in the hope of becoming a steadfast practitioner, faithful to the traditional martial art of taekwondo.

The Practice of Purpose in Taekwondo

In the summer of 1999, during a training excursion to Korea, Grandmaster Richard Chun and I were traveling south to Kyongju by bus along with a sizable contingent of our students. This offered me a wonderful opportunity to sit with my teacher and seek answers to questions we seldom had time to explore back home. After covering the obvious quandaries regarding history and culture, I decided to venture into less familiar territory. At the time I was faced with a dilemma that only someone with his vast experience could conceivably help me with. While the majority of martial arts schools across the nation are composed mainly of children, mine is disproportionately dominated by teens and adults. I wanted to know how I could provide my adult students with a challenging training experience while at the same time maintaining a reasonable and safe level of technical expectation.

In retrospect, Grandmaster Chun answered as I suspected and secretly hoped he would. He first stressed that all practitioners of taekwondo, regardless of age, should exhibit a strong spirit during training. This means, among other things, kihoping at the proper time, showing respect for seniors, and approaching class with a determined state of mind.[32] He also mentioned that ho sin sool techniques should be performed slowly and with great care so as to avoid any chance of injury. This advice was further tempered by the thought that the mature student should practice extreme caution when attempting to execute aerial, spinning, or jump turning kicks with the possibility, in some cases, of eliminating them altogether in favor of techniques less stressful on the body. These techniques, he intimated, would become less important in the promotion of a practitioner with the advancement of age. He reminded me that prior to sport-sparring, the front, round, and side kicks were the three basic tools of the art. While I saw the value in my grandmaster's words, I was, admittedly, a little confused. Shouldn't I be setting a single standard against which all are indiscriminately measured? As an instructor, how could I expect a certain level of proficiency from one segment of my student population while exempting another based solely on age?

"I am not suggesting that you compromise your standards," said Grandmaster Chun. "I am saying to hold your mature students to a slightly different, yet equally stringent standard. That standard," he continued, "is the demonstration of *purpose.*" Purpose here can be defined as an action signaled by controlled, mindful martial intent involving little or no contact. Immediately, a bulb switched on in my head as I became enlightened by my mentor's train of thought.

The practice of traditional taekwondo is composed of a variety of elements where the concept of purpose can be applied. Turning again to self-defense techniques, for example, the martial artist need not rush through a given procedure in order to test its effectiveness. Smooth, elegant, and purposeful motions will accomplish the same goal with fewer struggles since balance and simplicity are essential. Utilizing the body's pressure points located on the various anatomical meridians is another method to amplify technique without relying on excessive force.[33]

The same can be said for the ritualistic practice of one-, two-, and three-step sparring. When defending against an attack such as a reverse punch, the practitioner must assume that a block executed with purpose can potentially have the same result as a strike, rendering any additional countermeasure unnecessary. Kicking and punching drills, too, must contain an abundant supply of purpose. Simply because mature practitioners cannot deliver a round kick to the head region should not label them as incapable of defending themselves. On the contrary, a well-placed in-step round kick to the back of the thigh, practiced with mindful intent, should adequately incapacitate any attacker long enough to ensure escape. But perhaps the most important area where the application of purpose is most evident is in the performance of poomsae.

Formal patterns contain the words and syllables that compose the sentences of traditional taekwondo. From the initial motion to the segue between movements there is ample opportunity to apply the doctrine of purpose—show the block, project the strike, and follow through with the joint-lock or sweep. Do not simply step through the motions. That is dance, not martial arts.

We must recall that traditional taekwondo is democratic in nature. That is, its rewards and virtues are accessible to all regardless of age, gender, or physique. Therefore, rather than approach a particular technique in a half-hearted manner when shadowed by the specter of age, we must remember to add an ingredient of purpose into every stance, block, or strike we execute, imbuing it instead with meaning and mindful martial intent. Young or old, purpose and technical prowess are what we are promoted on.

And so, as our bus rolled closer and closer to our destination, my questions were meaningfully answered by a great teacher, a legend who has dedicated his life to traditional taekwondo. As an instructor, what better example could I have than Grandmaster Richard Chun? I recall thinking at the time of the good fortune that led me to become an instructor of taekwondo. Still, teaching martial arts is not the same as training in the martial arts. What drives students to become worthy instructors? What must they sacrifice in order to reap the rewards teaching brings?

The Calling

It is often said that "those who cannot do, teach." While this proverb may be true in some vocations, it does not necessarily apply to the martial arts. Even though proficiency in taekwondo is not automatically pegged to age, stories abound of elderly grandmasters far outdistancing their charges in aptitude based on years of experience and dedication to their art. Morihei Ueshiba, known to disciples of aikido as O Sensei, was said to have successfully battled several strong combatants simultaneously in his twilight years. Grandmaster Jhoon Rhee, the father of American taekwondo, trains while routinely performing hundreds of push-ups daily. The blocks and strikes demonstrated by Grandmaster Richard Chun during black belt seminars are awe-inspiring to watch while the same can be said for those of Grandmaster Gyoo Hyun Lee when teaching at his World Taekwondo Instructor Academy in South Korea.

What is it that induces men and women to forego the apparent comforts and entitlements sanctioned by age in favor of disciplined training? Often it is an intuitive sense that destiny has consigned them the role of becoming the repository of an ancient art, rich in philosophy, that must be passed on with honor and dignity in order to preserve its effectiveness and vitality. Very few

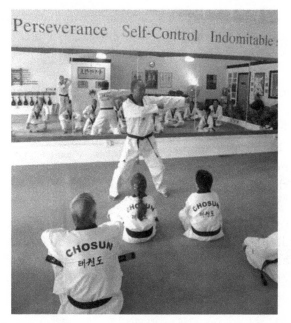

For decades, Grandmaster Richard Chun has answered the call to teach traditional taekwondo with enthusiasm and integrity.

individuals possess the spiritual stamina to answer this call with even fewer capable of enduring its hardships since they must realize that, as with any sincere pedagogical quest, financial gain is not the primary focus. This is not to say that the rewards are few. On the contrary, becoming an untarnished link in the great chain of martial arts knowledge, coupled with the ability to influence many lives in a positive manner through the transmission of a classical martial art, is frequently compensation enough for those who respond to the calling.

Yet it is a fact of life that the professional martial arts instructor must fiscally provide for self and family so as to enjoy a modicum of comfort within the bounds of today's society. And here a critical dichotomy exists; the school owner must walk a razor's edge between offering virtuous instruction and building commercial success. The martial arts professional is routinely assaulted by marketing companies charging monthly membership fees and putting clever labels on courses most martial arts schools should be providing anyway. These programs are useful for the instructor who has little to no business or marketing experience. They can hold sway by putting dollar signs over tradition. Still, if the instructor applies his efforts wholeheartedly to this noble pursuit in a sincere and benevolent fashion, potential and existing students will take notice and a comfortable level of monetary gain should follow.

But money, regardless of its lure, clearly is not the singular fuel that drives those destined to teach. Integrity, too, is largely a motivating force not simply because an instructor is expected to act as a role model for his students, but in a sense that traditional taekwondo must be passed on without distortion, gross personal interpretation, or corruption by foreign styles, leaving it, instead, pure for those who follow. As metaphysical as this may sound, a worthy instructor realizes the awesome responsibility that this

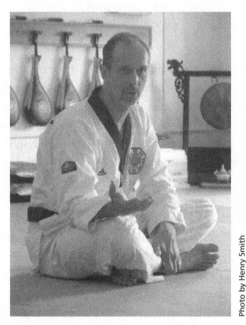

Photo by Henry Smith

The author describes himself as a link in the great chain of martial arts knowledge.

entails and appreciates his or her special place in the universal order.

Furthermore, a unique character is required to successfully embrace this calling. The *sabumnim* must develop an indomitable spirit while exhibiting the ability to efficiently motivate students of mixed skills to achieve extraordinary ends. Given the tenuous nature of the martial relationship, he must strive for balance, since the kinship that develops between a master and student of the martial arts is unlike any other that exists in everyday life. The depth of this alliance can fall anywhere between a passing acquaintance and prolonged discipleship. Attributes such as humility and compassion are essential since the instructor may be called upon to fill many roles. At times he may act as a counselor, confidant, spiritual advisor, parent figure, and, in certain situations, friend. The teacher is the guide, example, and focal point of the student's martial arts training. So as not to take this bond too lightly, the instructor must recall the foundation on which it is built. In spite of the prominent philosophical component of taekwondo, the martial arts, by definition, are based on a militaristic way of thinking; seniority, discipline, and rank all come into play, reflecting Asian cultural tradition as a whole. As well as assuming the role of benefactor, the master instructor can, at times, appear tyrannical, demanding, and, in extreme cases, masochistic. This potentially mercurial behavior is a direct result of the implied responsibilities that exist in the ever-evolving relationship between the student and the master.

Conversely, since the master instructor often sacrifices his own training time in favor of teaching and since the two are exclusive of one another, he must subjugate ego in attempting to further his own martial arts skills. An essential element of Buddhist thought is the realization that *the journey is more important than the destination* in tandem with that of *beginner's mind*. Taking these principles into consideration the competent instructor should seek the direction of one more accomplished than he if such an individual is readily available. At minimum, he should train consistently in the little time available, in a constant endeavor to retain exemplary proficiency. Technique should be nurtured and cherished just as should any treasured entity. It is not enough to simply possess technical skill; the instructor must acquire academic knowledge and cultivate internal strength through Ki development as well.

Regardless of title, whether it is sabumnim, sensei, or sifu, the instructor holds the future of the practitioner's martial life, quite literally, in his hands. His students are living reflections of the virtues he exemplifies. They echo his physical technique as well as the philosophical and spiritual values he espouses. Through strength he teaches discipline; through humility, compassion; through encouragement, self-esteem. He shares a common bond with teachers of the past in accepting with integrity a noble calling. In the end, the instructor has the awesome responsibility of passing on a martial tradition that he has personally refined in some small way, leaving his mark for future generations of martial artists to come.

Finally, in conjunction with the many talents the instructor must possess to effectively transmit martial arts skills, he must also possess *wisdom*—the wisdom to accept traditional taekwondo in its entirety so that nothing in the core curriculum is eliminated, ignored, or corrupted. And there is much to embrace.

The Holistic Acceptance of Taekwondo

Over the years, I have discovered that some practitioners approach the principles of the martial arts as they would a menu at a restaurant, making one selection from column "A" and another from column "B." This outlook is particularly common among newcomers and those who have not been exposed to, or genuinely embrace, the philosophical underpinnings of traditional taekwondo. In everyday jargon this habit is called "cherry-picking" and while it may work in food, fashion, and farming, it does not work in the sincere study of taekwondo. Korean martial arts doctrine can be viewed as a complex puzzle composed of many ideas foreign to the Western mind. Selectively removing or ignoring any of these concepts for whatever reason significantly reduces the value of traditional taekwondo training.

The martial arts are intrinsically tied to the three Asian philosophical paradigms of Buddhism, Taoism, and Confucianism. Each of these in its own way has contributed greatly to the fertile ground that nurtures the seeds of discovery and enlightenment exclusive to taekwondo. The training process, physically, spiritually, and mentally, will bear fruit only if the practitioner permits nature and the wisdom inherent in these ancient ideals to run their course. Just as an apple will not ripen properly if picked too early, or worse, die on the tree if exposed to pollutants in the soil, so the taekwondoist will suffer if the principles that separate the martial arts from a common lifestyle are conveniently discounted or overlooked altogether.

Let us take, for example, something as deceptively simple as the bow of courtesy so ubiquitous in traditional taekwondo. I say "deceptively simple" because on the surface, an uninitiated onlooker merely sees two individuals inclining their upper bodies at a precise angle toward one another. Undoubtedly, the bow, which replaces the handshake in many parts of the world, holds obvious salutary value. However, we as martial artists realize that there is much more to this action than meets the eye. Aside from a demonstration of respect, the bow, *kyungye* in Korean, represents a myriad of implied principles, principles that must be upheld if taekwondo is ever to survive in a classical form. Bowing to a fellow student represents an acknowledgement that the techniques we practice can be lethal if abused and therefore must be wielded with self-control. Likewise, bowing to a master instructor is not only an expression of respect and humility, but an essential sign of loyalty unhindered by outside influences. In reciprocity, the master instructor is silently communicating to his students that he will watch over them and do his best in helping them navigate the often confusing journey through taekwondo, however severe he may seem. An instructor bowing to a fellow instructor not only implies mutual respect, but that they will treat one another with honor in their relationship. Lastly, bowing at the threshold of the dojang before entering is yet another manifestation of the student's appreciation for the holistic practice of traditional taekwondo. This simple gesture recognizes the spiritual boundary that separates the routine of everyday life from the supercharged atmosphere of the dojang, the sacred place where we come to study *The Way*. Given the depth of this gesture, how could anyone fail to formally acknowledge the virtues that are portrayed?

Vocal cues, too, hold special significance to those who practice taekwondo in its fullness. In an effort to minimize the loss of students due to an overt demand for discipline, some schools have eliminated the required reply of "Yes, Sir" or "Yes, Ma'am" that is spoken by a junior when addressing a senior student or instructor. Even the spirit yell, or kihop, that is so vitally needed to amplify a strike, block, or kick, is often overlooked and rendered unnecessary.

Similarly, the exclusion of meditation, Ki development exercises, basic technique practice, self-defense drills, and most urgently, poomsae, from the standard curriculum due to a strong emphasis on sport competition, has a devastating effect on the student's overall maturity as a complete martial artist. All of these omissions eat away at the very foundation of traditional taekwondo leaving less and less to pass on to future generations.

For the most part, the ideology of taekwondo when practiced as a classical martial art has been forged in the fires of Asian culture. Naturally, practitioners in the West often find this worldview difficult to conceptualize. For instance, once while training in Korea I recall seeing an instructor strike a student with a kicking target because he felt the student was not performing up to par.[34] In that setting the teacher's punitive action was not construed as being cruel or unusual. Training for eight hours at a time, as we did, in a dojang with interior temperatures of ninety degrees or more, is commonplace in Korea and elicits not a word of criticism. I provide these experiences for consideration not because I necessarily support them, but because they unmistakably drive home the point that there are fundamental differences in the way local training is taught as compared to the manner in which it is practiced in Korea, taekwondo's country of origin. To complain about an instructor in Korea is unthinkable. To question his authority is worse. Behavior of this nature is not unique to taekwondo but represents a microcosm of Korean society at large. It is neither right nor wrong; it simply *is* and stems from the hierarchal societal structure embedded in Confucian thought.

Metaphorically speaking, if we wish to truly absorb the culture of a nation, we must attempt to speak the language, eat the food, dress accordingly, and conform to local customs. The same guidelines hold true for traditional taekwondo; we must accept its physical component, mental requirements, and spiritual principles as a whole—without condition.

Clearly, the complete and sincere practice of taekwondo is not for everyone. In order to achieve excellence in our training, we must suppress our individual selves, bend to seniority, practice diligently and without complaint, remain loyal to style and school, and finally, act with honor in establishing an enduring trust between teacher and student. Remaining steadfast to these seemingly unreachable ideals does not require a character of super-eminent proportions; rather, it demands a noble heart and an unswerving love for the martial arts that only those willing to accept traditional taekwondo in its entirety will be successful in developing. I have been fortunate over the course of my training to become acquainted with many inspirational individuals who have epitomized these ideals not only in their physical acceptance of the art, but also in their ability to rise above hardship. All could have easily surrendered to adversity but intentionally did not. Let us meet some of them now.

Champions of the Heart

The philosophical component of the *I Ching* that corresponds to WTF poomsae Taegeuk Sa Jang represents thunder. Thunder, along with the lightning and noise that accompanies it, evokes fear and trembling but reminds us that adversity, like a thunderstorm, can pass as suddenly as it arrives, leaving blue sky, sunshine, and rain-freshened air in its wake. Subsequently, if performed with mindful intent, this form along with its underlying philosophy, teaches the martial artist to face adversity with courage if he or she is to prevail. How does this ornate but promising description apply to daily life?

Adversity comes in many flavors. Clearly, it can materialize bundled in with health or money matters that have spun out of control. However, on a more benign level, yet equally as immediate, adversity can manifest itself in challenges to our taekwondo training. Not long ago, a group of colleagues and I were faced with a situation that required a collective, yet highly individual, approach to resolve. The players affected by this situation are, and will remain, true "Champions of the Heart," humble, yet tenacious in their pursuit of traditional taekwondo.

Our story begins during a time when a school that had existed for over forty years under the leadership of a renowned grandmaster changed hands. I, along with a group of black belts ranging in rank from 1st to 6th dan, trained there on a weekly basis. Regrettably, the new owner, either by choice or through ignorance, began teaching an aerobic-oriented, mixed martial arts curriculum rather than continuing with the syllabus rich in traditional taekwondo technique for which the previous institution had become world famous.

Remaining on during the transition, the head instructor, Paul, a 6th dan, became embroiled in a disagreement with management and with great disappointment left suddenly after teaching for nearly two decades at the same location. While the new owner kindly allowed the majority of us to congregate and train, we increasingly found ourselves segregated from the main body of students while practicing forms, kicking, and self-defense drills on our own. Clearly, due to space limitations, this could not continue for long and one by one, we left in frustration, concerned about the future of our training and the traditions we hoped to protect.

Then one day I received a telephone call from a 5th dan who had also attended our old school. Sam, a highly capable instructor, was not only my senior, but a mentor and, thankfully, my long-time training partner. In a shocking disclosure, he confided to me that he had suffered a minor heart ailment and would be out of commission for at least six months. Assured that his condition was past the critical stage, we both expressed regret that our mutual practice would be temporarily curtailed.

As the months went by, I continued training daily with my students at the Chosun Taekwondo Academy. Still, I missed the honor and opportunity to work with my seniors. Occasionally, I would call Sam to check on his condition. Meanwhile, Paul, I discovered, was recovering from a long-overdue hip replacement. With this news came what I thought was the final dissolution of our original group and the end of a long and rewarding training experience.

More time passed and I began to hear a rumor that Paul had begun teaching at a new location following a complete recovery from his surgery. I was delighted when he invited me to visit and train. However, as fate would have it, my teaching responsibilities made it difficult for me to break away and make the four-hour roundtrip to New York City. Then Sam called and said that his physician had given him permission to resume training. This, I felt, was a favorable omen and, undeterred, I told him I would meet him the very next week at the dojang where Paul was teaching.

A few days later, after parking my car, I strolled down First Avenue in the direction of the training hall. The holiday spirit had descended on New York and the streets were a riot of colorful lights accented by the scent of pine that lingered in the air from the Christmas trees being sold on almost every corner. I opened the main door of a private school that housed the dojang owned by Amanda, an outstanding martial artist who charitably welcomed us in our time of need, and with anticipation I bolted down a short flight of stairs two at a time.[35] There, among a group of practitioners, stood Paul, looking fit as ever. It had been

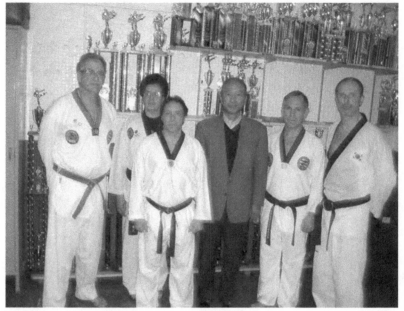

Photo by Henry Smith

Training at Haddock Taekwondo, New York City (left to right) Masters Samuel Mizrahi, Amanda Haddock, Pablo Alejandro, Grandmaster Richard Chun, Maurice Elmalem, and Doug Cook.

some time since last we met, and following a friendly embrace, he invited me onto the mat. Before long, Sam appeared along with yet another black belt who had trained with us previously. Looking around as Paul shouted *"Cha Riot!"* I could not believe my eyes—the bulk of us together again after a year of independent practice. Following a dynamic two-hour class, with perspiration burning my eyes, I thought how easy it would have been a few short months ago for any one of us to surrender to defeat. Yet here we were: Paul, recovering from orthopedic surgery; Sam, living in the shadow of a potentially-tragic cardiac event; all of us licking our wounds from the loss of a school. This time, adversity and doubt had taken a back seat to courage and tenacity. Indomitable spirit ruled. These fine martial artists could easily have fallen back on the excuse of being physically incapable of continuing intense training. Instead, here was Sam executing a jump spinning crescent kick, his signature technique, with more grace and power than ever before. Did his illness represent a catharsis rather than a setback? And Paul, again throwing head-level round kicks that a short while ago were seriously impeded by chronic injury. Rather than being frustrated by an extended recovery, both these gentlemen were vigorously pushing the limits of excellence. In that dojang, on that evening, before my eyes rose a Phoenix of the soul. A banner could have been raised in celebration with words emblazoned:

Here Train Champions of the Heart,
Steadfast Conquerors of Thunder:
The Men and Women of Traditional Taekwondo

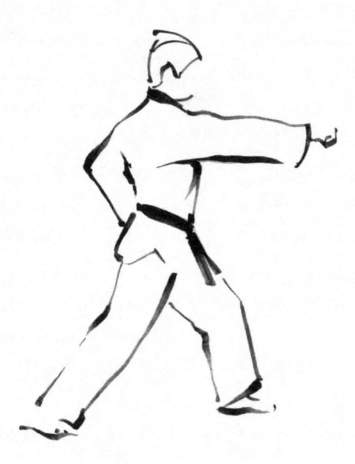

Part Four

Just for Beginners

First Steps

The most difficult part of traditional taekwondo is not learning the first kick or punch. It is not struggling to remember the motions of a poomsae or becoming acquainted with Korean culture. Rather, it is taking the first step across the threshold of the dojang door. This is a point where roads diverge, where choices are made that will resonate throughout a lifetime.

Without a doubt, most students reflect on their first days of training with memories of apprehension, wonder, anticipation, and accomplishment: apprehension based on the mostly unfounded fear of potential injury, wonder at the potent secrets hidden within the martial arts, anticipation at the vast landscape of possibilities they represent, and, ultimately, accomplishment in the sense that they have persevered long enough to overcome the myriad challenges endured by the novice. Just like a cork riding up and down on a troubled sea, all martial artists, at one time or another, experience self-doubt mixed with exhilaration and tedium commingled with enthusiasm. However, since taekwondo practice mirrors life, shifts in behavior are to be expected. With this in mind, an ingredient of self-moderation must be cultivated in an effort to balance extremes in temperament. These are lessons sincere taekwondoists will carry with them day and night, year in, year out as they come to realize that traditional taekwondo is a way of life and not a seasonal pursuit as is sport.

As a color belt, students can effectively visualize themselves as hovering above a great globe of knowledge. Upon earning the black belt, they barely skim the surface of this complex world. With each successive year of practice, the student drills down ever closer to the core of taekwondo. This takes a brand of patience uncommon in modern society. Yet this persistence, this ability to endure, nurtures a unique, mindful character so essential in dealing with the adversities of daily life. Subsequently, just as basic technique, forms, and sparring—the vital elements of traditional taekwondo—represent the *physical* bedrock of the art, psychological defensive strategies, too, can be cultivated in an effort to fortify the mind. These life lessons are of great value to students wanting to gain a profound understanding of the martial arts and what they mean to the individual in the twenty-first century.

Enduring Strength

The world today is a complex and demanding place filled with reward, sacrifice, and adversity. We are born into the lives we lead and deserve nothing more than what we gain through honest work. Some believe that in order to get ahead they must think first and foremost of themselves. While destiny may be fulfilled by the actions we channel toward our quest for personal success, both in our martial arts training and in private pursuits, we must also develop a compassionate heart and remain sensitive to the needs of others. Perhaps most important, we must cultivate *enduring strength,* the strength necessary to protect ourselves and our clarity of mind from extreme adversity. Enduring strength can further be quantified as the psychological muscle required to abide radical pain and suffering whether it be unique to the individual or external in nature relating to someone we know and love. It is the ability to remain focused regardless of intense distraction in order to provide support and stability to those around us at a time when they may need it most. Often it is irrelevant whether the trouble is physically or mentally rooted since the despair it creates results in the same emotional distress. Exhibiting enduring strength may begin by merely acting the part, putting on a game face and attempting not to waver while, in reality, your soul is plagued with fear. This may be a very difficult task to accomplish particularly if the crisis has come as a shock or surprise.

Fortunately, traditional taekwondo provides a platform upon which enduring strength can be nurtured. However, being a martial artist does not automatically qualify the practitioner as being someone gifted with enduring strength. On the contrary, having shed the bravado many people artificially display in trying times, we as taekwondoists, by virtue of the humility demanded by diligent training, appreciate the great effort required to genuinely develop the simplest component of a strong character. Yet our ability to remain open to change and self-improvement gives us a leg up in our attempt to generate what amounts to internal resiliency. Furthermore, to realize the virtue of enduring strength, martial artists must approach their training with sincerity and purpose, fully appreciating the value of *do*, or *The Way* . Mindful practice of any classical martial way assumes that the practitioner is intent on a path toward holistic enrichment and not just in search of combat skills. Paradoxically, it is through the practice of these combat skills that the martial artist nurtures moral fiber.

Regrettably, turmoil frequently lingers, causing enduring strength to float on a foundation of patience. Sickness, financial strain, and family unrest have no determinate timetable, forcing the individual to undergo seemingly unremitting stress and confusion. However, martial artists devoted to their practice can testify to the fact that patience is the cornerstone of progress. The waiting period between color belt, or *gup* levels, is clearly an exercise in patience while the time span between dan, or black belt degree levels, is decidedly measured in years. This custom of waiting cultivates undeniable patience that can be transferred to any situation in life.[36]

If the practitioner is following the path of traditional taekwondo, then certainly meditation and its related benefits is a vital ingredient of his training regimen. There are many goals of meditation in the martial arts, but when attempting to build enduring strength, serenity of mind in conjunction with Ki enhancement is a major contributor. Sitting in quiet reflection for a period of fifteen minutes in the morning or evening can prove to be a potent elixir when faced with an unending deluge of anxiety. Likewise, the period of meditation can be used to visualize Ki, fortifying the mind and body against the demons of constant worry. The universal life force is not only an effective tool in amplifying combat technique, but in a practical sense, acts as a shield against bodily damage, positioning it as a worthy ally of enduring strength. Consequently, Ki not only *projects*, but *protects*.[37]

When examined closely, all aspects of taekwondo training can have a profound effect on the promotion of enduring strength. Something as basic as a solid front stance (*ap koobi*) when executed correctly, can have an enormous centering effect on the human psyche. Sparring, too, with its tendency to point out our strengths and weaknesses within the framework of a combat environment, fosters courage in the face of danger. Clearly, this is no small contribution when dealing with uninvited hardship.

Additionally, the breaking of solid objects or *kyuk pa,* while often viewed as the theatrical component of taekwondo, realistically develops focus and willpower. The destruction of a one-inch pine board by a determined taekwondoist is used to confirm the penetrating force of a punch or kick. Similarly, the mental energy required to conquer a seemingly unyielding situation in life requires the same sort of spirit and is mirrored by this act of indomitable will. Even the simple act, if it can be termed as such, of hard training enriches the senses through chemical reactions in the body leaving the martial artist refreshed and invigorated following an intense class.

The classical martial arts offer support for enduring strength when viewed from their various philosophical perspectives as well. Most forms of traditional training acknowledge the influence of Zen Buddhist doctrine. Plainly put, one of the key elements of this spiritual paradigm is the principle of existing in the here and now. This permits the practitioner to appreciate the moment in its fullness rather than becoming apprehensive about the future or concerned with the past. If approached in this manner, the specter of misfortune can be relegated to a place on the periphery of our consciousness rather than permitting it to assume center stage in our daily routine, consuming us with worry. By the same token, Taoism teaches us that *everything occurs in its appointed time,* and as clinical as this notion may initially appear when seeking solace from unbearable, emotional pain, it does presume a grand design outside the current scope of our understanding. Remaining focused and devoted to traditional taekwondo training often results in the distraction the victim needs most when dealing with difficult times. In a therapeutic sense, while intense practice may not be the decisive answer to every problem, it represents a lifeboat on a sea of troubled waters.

At some point in our lives we must accept the necessity of defending ourselves when terrifying emotional stress or physical danger surfaces. Life is not exclusively Yang, but Um as well, often jubilant but in darker times, less forgiving. How we deal with this dichotomy dictates the quality of our existence. It is the goal of the martial artist, especially those cognizant of *The Way,* to live life to its fullest as defined by the individual.

Enduring strength, the worthy adversary of extreme adversity, is yet another hardened tool to be used in our quest for self-realization through the martial arts. However, before any psychological defense can be mustered, we must first remain open to suggestion while *surrendering* any preconceived notions in the process.

Surrender!

After teaching taekwondo for many years, I have come to some concrete observations. As an instructor and school owner I have noticed that many new students have a difficult time acclimating to Eastern customs. Certainly this is understandable given the difference in worldview between Asian culture and ours in the West. What is the remedy to this dilemma? How does the competent instructor motivate students to remain, following their first

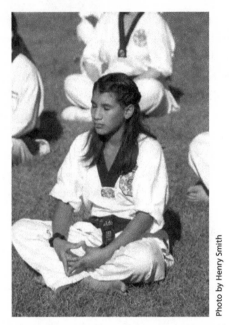

Photo by Henry Smith

Surrender, through meditation, promotes a tranquil mind.

few classes, in order to reap the benefits of long-term martial arts training?

The good news is that a silver bullet *does* exist in response to this quandary and the answer is—*Surrender!* Yes, before any new information or skill—of whatever nature—can be absorbed, the individual must clear the mind, wipe clean the mental blackboard, and empty the cup. All existing preconceptions concerning the martial arts need to be released—in essence, *surrendered*. This principle, if applied consistently, will not only act as a remedy for many initial misapprehensions, but over time, will result in more rewarding training sessions both physically and mentally.

For instance, the required bow of respect that is part and parcel of taekwondo etiquette causes some to go scurrying from the training hall before the first kick is ever thrown. Add to this the practice of meditation coupled with Ki development exercises—techniques that resonate with metaphysics—and what is often left is a recipe for a quick departure. In my school, for example, the population is composed primarily of adults; issues such as flexibility, stamina, age, gender, and memory all come into play.

Behavioral patterns ingrained since childhood find men and women, particularly in the formative stages of their training, relating differently to taekwondo instruction. By way of example, having been involved in schoolyard squabbles as an adolescent, the adult male often feels that he is experienced in the ways of combat. Additionally, having observed fight scenes on television and in the cinema, many men come equipped with baggage that needs to be replaced with authentic defensive skills supported by an appreciation for the damage they inflict. Another fundamental impediment is the male ego that is expressed as a tendency to fear the appearance of ignorance regardless of subject matter.

Women, on the other hand, face a different sort of challenge. Many adult females who practice taekwondo do so with their family and are, therefore, mothers. Performing a deadly counterattack on an adversary clearly bent on bodily harm presents the likelihood of triggering a maternal instinct that reminds the defender that she is about to injure someone else's child regardless of intent. This unfortunate situation is certain to result in a flicker of response time with possibly fatal consequences. And then there is the overriding embarrassment of women being subconsciously programmed over countless years by society in general to be both timid and subservient. Observe a novice adult woman's fighting, or as I more correctly refer to it, a defense stance; the guard hand is often drawn in close to the woman's body in an almost obvious refusal to claim the immediate space around her that is her birthright.

Certainly, there are other obstacles we can identify that hinder the painless acceptance of martial arts decorum and technique. Yet these roadblocks to progress must be removed if we expect to enjoy a rewarding training experience. What is the remedy to this dilemma? Again, Surrender!

Let us for a moment examine how this notion of surrender can be applied during a typical taekwondo class. The student arrives at the dojang after a busy day at school or work. The mind is ripe with distractions, the body fatigued from physical stress. The session begins with a period of meditation. Surrender to the moment. Think of the mind as a glass of water drawn from a pond containing a quantity of sediment. Allowing the glass to sit undisturbed for a moment will permit the particles to settle causing the liquid to clear. The same holds true of the mind. With some effort, surrendering all concerns to the task at hand will prepare the mind to not only accept new information without being distracted, but will set the stage for more focused training.

Next, muscles taut from sitting at a desk all day or riding in a car must be permitted to relax safely. During flexibility exercises, students should breathe into the particular stretch and not hold their breath. They should also visualize the muscles elongating with each exhalation and, literally, surrender to the stretch.

As the core curriculum continues focusing on basics, poomsae, and self-defense, it is a simple matter for students to compare themselves to each other—particularly low belts to advanced belts, adults to teens. Being overly judgmental of their technique can create a highly toxic situation. Better to leave self-criticism on the doorstep and simply—do. Dwelling on how poorly a kick was executed or, conversely, congratulating yourself on a poomsae well done will interfere with the natural flow of technique. Instead, dismiss conscious self-evaluation and surrender to an empty mind as described in the practice of Zen meditation. Personally, some of my most memorable training experiences involved the conscious dismissal of self-judgment.

Lastly, the practice of free-sparring can offer yet another opportunity to utilize the gift of surrender. In order to act rapidly in competition or in the face of a true threat that has escalated beyond verbal mediation, the mind in concert with the body must *react* rather than *anticipate*. Making the false assumption that an opponent will execute a reverse punch when, in truth, his intention is to kick may result in severe injury to the defender, or at best, a point in favor of the opponent. To appreciate the value of surrender, the concept of *mushin*, or mind/no mind, the mental condition that frees the spirit of preconceived notions and expectations during practice should be applied as well.

Many of the scenarios examined here relate to the experienced practitioner. Those standing at the threshold of the martial arts would do well to release all prejudice concerning decorum and simply appreciate the cultural relevancy of the act they are performing along with the philosophical underpinnings in which they are rooted. Bowing clearly does not make one a slave to another, nor does vigorously responding "Yes, Sir" or "Yes, Ma'am" to a command. Likewise, admitting that a body of knowledge is radically and, for that matter, literally foreign in nature does not label you as being incompetent. On the contrary, having the courage to pursue a discipline steeped in honor and tradition demonstrates your ability to embrace exciting, new concepts in life unencumbered by the fear of appearing inept.

For all these reasons, traditional taekwondo practice is as relevant today as it was decades ago and, in some cases, even more so. Yet enrichment of character, as the suffix *do* in taekwondo implies, comes at a cost. But in order to realize the benefits of disciplined training in its fullness, both the novice and experienced practitioner alike must remember to *surrender* to new concepts and methods on their path to self-enrichment. Understandably, demonstrating the resilience to make judgment calls of this nature often results in untoward emotional stress complicating practice even further. And here we are faced with a question: Is the intensity of stress commonly generated by traditional taekwondo training necessarily detrimental? Or is it something to be acknowledged, respected, and ultimately confronted in the same manner as would an accommodating training partner in learning how to conquer chronic stress in daily life.

Stress in the Martial Arts

Stress for taekwondoists can be defined as a function of the expectations we impose upon ourselves in response to a challenge. This is why I often find it comical when martial arts schools unequivocally promise the hope of stress-reduction in their advertisements. Certainly there is something to be said about the release you feel when punching and kicking targets after a particularly trying day. Working up a good sweat as endorphins course through the bloodstream is undoubtedly a potent elixir for blowing off steam, but represents the extent to which many busy people are willing to go in an effort to purge pent up anxiety. Admittedly, schools flying the martial arts banner focus on this type of physically-intensive program with great commercial success. However, the aerobic workout you receive during a class of this nature reflects only a small portion of the traditional taekwondo curriculum. The sign over the door of these establishments should more accurately read something along the line of Kick Aerobics or Tae Boxing rather than Taekwondo.

At this point it should be noted that anything worth doing has the potential of producing a modicum of stress, which comes in many flavors and just as in the case of good and bad cholesterol, there is good and bad stress. For instance, the tension students recall experiencing during their first date is significantly different from the anxiety that is part and parcel of a visit to the dentist. Likewise, the anticipation we feel prior to leaving for an extended vacation is different from the frustration that frequently accompanies living with our in-laws! Challenges that stimulate the mind, body, and spirit, while forever elevating the consciousness of the individual, can generate an entirely different brand of stress. Attaining the peak of some great mountain, giving the perfect musical performance, publishing a book, receiving a doctorate, and, yes, earning a black belt through the sincere study of traditional taekwondo, all fall into this category, proof positive that quests rewarded by a great sense of achievement routinely exact their cost and take their toll.

Clearly, for those seeking nothing more from their training than an adrenaline-filled, heart pumping workout, the stress relief associated with a martial-oriented aerobics program is instantly gratifying but leaves the spiritual and philosophical components of the martial *arts* largely ignored. Yet there are those noble few who seek authenticity in parallel with self-enrichment through the practice of traditional taekwondo regardless of the depth and complexity of the challenges presented.

Take, for instance, the performance of poomsae, which represents the essence of traditional taekwondo or any classical martial art for that matter. No doubt, learning a new form, refining it, and memorizing its tactical intent can be a demanding enterprise particularly if it is taken seriously and approached with diligence. Multiply this challenge by the number of poomsae a black belt is expected to possess, regardless of heritage, and you can appreciate the level of stress associated with this prospect. Think of it: A 1st dan WTF-stylist may be expected to perform the three *Kicho* forms in conjunction with the eight Taegeuk, eight Palgwe, and the required Koryo, at a moment's notice. Likewise, an ITF practitioner of equivalent rank is obligated to execute tul, or patterns, ranging from *Chon-Ji* to *Ge-Baek* and beyond. In truth, students training at my dojang, the Chosun Taekwondo Academy, are expected to be proficient at the *Pyung-Ahn* series, the *Kibon* set, and a number of Moo Duk Kwan black belt poomsae in addition to those mentioned above. In total, this can be as many as thirty-two forms, yet if practiced on a weekly basis it is more than possible to recall them all when necessary. Miss a few classes, however, and a profound sense of incompetence, mixed with the embarrassment an erroneous performance can produce, invariably conjures up a serving of stress many find debilitating.

If the practice of formal patterns is not enough to cause the practitioner sufficient anguish, then there are the limitless concerns inherent in the memorization and proper execution of one-step sparring and self-defense drills. "Do I step back with my right leg or my left?" or "What stance am I in?" or "Do I block with a single or double knife hand technique?"[38] As a professional instructor, I regularly observe confusion in the faces of students who either lead very busy lives that prohibit consistent attendance or have entered the dojang with a heavy mind brimming over with distractions. Regardless of the cause, the stress produced by situations such as these is symptomatic of the challenges involved and the expectations of meeting these challenges.

Clearly, most people who study traditional taekwondo truly desire to do their best in practice and for the most part, they do. Still, there are mutual obligations involved on both sides of the equation, between the student and the instructor, which must be respected particularly if measurable progress is to be realized and the stress connected with this advancement maintained at a manageable level. The symmetry of this relationship should flow along these lines: If the student is truly committed to his or her training and attempts to attend as many classes as reasonably possible within the framework of a hectic lifestyle, then the instructor must approach the situation with compassion, providing the practitioner with a limited amount of technique at each training session. In return, the student should practice remotely and return to class in full possession of the previously learned lessons so that his training may advance, albeit at a slower pace. Motivating a student to continue training in this manner should attenuate the stress that would otherwise escalate cumulatively, resulting in a decision to terminate training all together.

Other tranquilizing elements exist that can act as remedies in the fight against burnout due to self-imposed stress in the martial arts: eliminating self-judgment, the toxic trait that causes you to over-analyze technique relative to your performance, maintaining *beginner's mind*, the Zen state that encourages clarity and openness in the pursuit of daily life, and finally, mushin, or mind/ no mind. These psychological exercises, if applied sincerely, will allow the practitioner to *de-stress*, rather than *distress*.

Of course, this all assumes that one final ingredient is present that acts as a catalyst in compounding success in the martial arts, and that is a deep and lasting love for taekwondo down to its root. Without that, no amount of stress, good or bad, can be endured.

But why subject ourselves as martial artists to stress of an unnecessary nature that can be almost certainly eliminated in the first place? For instance, stress stemming from an ignorance of academic topics related to traditional taekwondo, such as Korean history, technical nomenclature, and even the basic requirements for a particular belt level, can be addressed as would any serious scholarly study. Enthusiastically taking notes and creating a comprehensive, written collection of knowledge in the form of a training journal is one solution.

Creating a Training Journal

The achievement of mind and body unification in traditional taekwondo is paramount for the realization of efficient technique. On one hand, the body must be conditioned to embrace strenuous training and dynamic skill foreign to ordinary motion. Conversely, the mind must remain open to the traditions, culture, and customs of Asian thought while simultaneously retaining vital, related information. Faithfully attending class on a daily basis stimulates the physical self to accurately repeat acquired skill. Yet how can the student fortify the mind to support the intellectual demands of traditional taekwondo?

Fortunately, textbooks and notebooks filled with hand-written information can still be found in schoolrooms and on college campuses around the globe, sharing the spotlight with laptops and Web sites alike. Without these classroom staples, learning would be difficult at best, if not impossible. Similarly, creating and maintaining a training journal containing the curriculum, experiences, and mementos unique to the student's practice of traditional taekwondo is an equally powerful instrument in the retention and retrieval of an individual's acquired knowledge. While it is difficult to gauge the expectations of various martial arts schools throughout the country, it has become a tradition in our dojang for students to create and maintain an all-inclusive, up-to-date training journal as a prerequisite for black belt and beyond. Indeed, students must present their personalized training journal to the examiner on the occasion of their black belt promotion test.

Composing a training journal is easy and enjoyable. Aside from providing practitioners with a complete picture of their training to date, it becomes a vehicle for reflecting on past accomplishments and experiences. To begin with, students need to acquire a three-ring loose-leaf binder with a transparent plastic sleeve on the front capable of holding a cover sheet. Through the wonder of computer graphics, students can use their imagination in generating a creative yet dignified cover. Clearly, the school logo and student name should prominently appear. All internal entries should be shielded by plastic page protectors. The journal is now ready to be filled with information divided according to belt rank. This can be accomplished using color paper corresponding to belt color or simply through the use of adhesive tabs. Curriculum sheets should comprise the core of the document, provided collateral material of this nature exists at the student's dojang. At the Chosun Taekwondo Academy, we adhere to a stringent curriculum composed of a repeating template that increases in complexity throughout the various belt levels; promotion from one rank to the next is predicated on proficiency in an escalating series of basics, one-step sparring, self-defense drills, poomsae, sparring, and breaking skills. Concurrently, students are expected

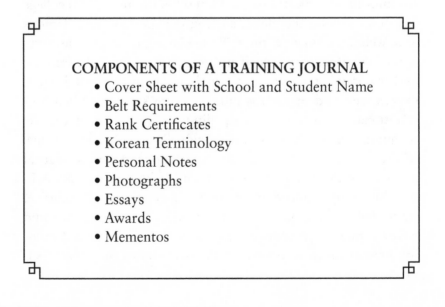

COMPONENTS OF A TRAINING JOURNAL
- Cover Sheet with School and Student Name
- Belt Requirements
- Rank Certificates
- Korean Terminology
- Personal Notes
- Photographs
- Essays
- Awards
- Mementos

to become acquainted with Korean history, terminology, and the philosophy associated with their poomsae. Everything is clearly written out to avoid confusion and presented to students to be included in their training journal. If a school does not provide this sort of documentation, then the student will need to create a repeatable outline that organizes this information in an orderly fashion according to belt rank.

Since the diligent practice of traditional taekwondo clearly contains an academic component, students who attend our dojang, as is the case with many schools, must submit a short essay in order to qualify for promotion.[39] Subjects vary according to the student's accumulated exposure to the martial arts. Writing an essay on a specified topic allows complicated concepts such as meditation, Ki development, and poomsae philosophy to become crystallized in the mind of the author. Given the amount of thought and effort invested in the composition of an essay, these too should be included in the training journal. Reviewing essays written in years past offers a rare and often surprising retrospective of a student's unique journey through the martial arts.

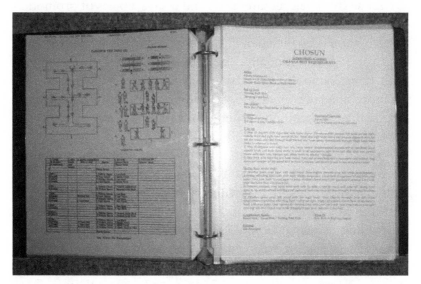

Training journal showing poomsae diagram and belt requirement sheet.

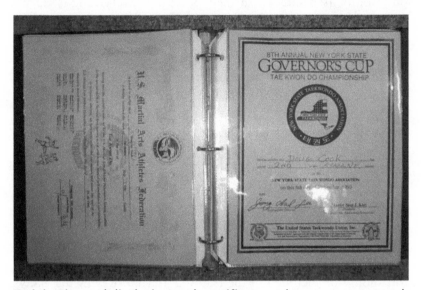

Training journal displaying rank certificate and tournament award.

Aside from belt requirements and essays, copies of promotion certificates and any competition, achievement, or recognition awards should be included in this practical repository of knowledge as well. Additionally, students often embellish their work with items symbolizing outstanding moments in their training. Memorabilia such as newspaper clippings and photographs add personality and color to an endeavor that can too quickly turn clinical in its approach.

Yet a journal by definition is a place to record innermost impressions, and this volume is no exception. For instance, the frustration associated with throwing the first round kick or the joy of performing a near-perfect poomsae promises to provide insightful reading in years to come.[40] Techniques offered during special training sessions are frequently not repeated in a standard class and should be captured in writing for future practice. And then there are gems of wisdom spoken by grandmasters that act as an elixir in granting solace when the training gets tough.

A training journal is an all-inclusive compendium of thoughts, documents, mementos, and valued lessons taught at the dojang. It is a way to organize a student's training between the covers of a book. It has the potential of lifting up that student and providing support when memory fails. Finally, it is crucial to begin compiling the journal early in the beginner's training rather than experience regret at the loss of information later on. Training journals geared toward children are commercially available while teens and adults must rely on originality, resolve, and painstaking attention to detail in order to create a volume worthy of the art.

We must remember that none of these time-honored martial traditions would be available to Westerners if the founders of the art had not made them accessible in the first place, initially through servicemen returning from Korea, and later on, through personal instruction around the world. While transmission of this knowledge was initially guarded due to its very nature, grandmasters today, for the most part, are eager to transmit their art to individuals deserving of their efforts. Finding a grandmaster with legitimate credentials, earning a place in his dojang, and faithfully conforming to his style of teaching is no easy chore given today's *McDojang* culture. Yet once the serious martial artist is successful in his or her quest, the benefits offered by this type of affiliation are priceless.

In the Shadow of a Grandmaster

I consider myself and the students I teach fortunate indeed, not simply because we are graced with a comfortable, clean, and culturally-focused training environment, but because we are members of an elite organization under the direction of a world-renowned grandmaster who promotes a traditional style of taekwondo.[41] In the modern world of mixed martial arts and schools boasting curricula "so simple a child can do it," we sometimes forget the value our type of heritage offers. The legacy our school enjoys not only reflects the comprehensive nature of taekwondo, but recognizes the individuals responsible for shepherding our discipline through its formative stages up to the present.

It is no secret that the roots of taekwondo were greatly influenced by Japanese Shotokan karate-do as well as various forms of Chinese fighting arts. And there currently exists a clear delineation between the traditional martial art of taekwondo and its sportive mate firmly based on Olympic-style sparring. Nevertheless, the present state of taekwondo as it applies to both the defensive art and world sport, coupled with the outstanding success it has achieved, is unquestionably linked to the masters and grandmasters native to the Korean peninsula that have refined and transmitted taekwondo's unique set of techniques and philosophical doctrines over the decades. Subsequently, maintaining a relationship with an elder instructor having a direct link to the founders of the art nurtures respect for heritage in tandem with technical accuracy—benefits that cannot be overstated.

Establishing a modern martial art based on the elements of other traditional disciplines may have its benefits as evidenced by the popularity of jeet kune do (way of the intercepting fist), the martial art created by the late Bruce Lee.[42] Yet, in today's age of Internet certification and canned curricula, it is far too easy to pick and choose techniques that highlight the physical abilities of an individual instructor, leaving out countless defensive strategies that require years to refine in the process. In many cases the long-range efficacy of these endeavors turns out to be suspect at best, causing students to question the authenticity of their art. Pitfalls such as this can be avoided by following in the footsteps of an experienced and legitimate grandmaster that supports a single combat-proven discipline based on heritage.

Training under a grandmaster, 7th dan or above, one that is an acknowledged source of traditional skills, is akin to being in possession of the original copy of an important document displaying clear and concise print. Undisputedly accurate in its current iteration, copies of this document, particularly those many generations later, are certain to diminish in quality resulting in distortion and possible misinterpretation. The same principle holds true

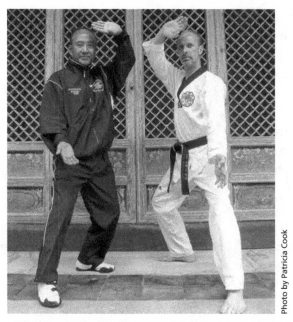

Photo by Patricia Cook

The author (right) with his mentor and teacher, Grandmaster Richard Chun, at Bulguksa Temple in South Korea.

when learning a kick, block, or strike. A simple twist of the wrist, turn of the hip, or snap of the leg, passed on by a human vessel with decades of experience can make the difference between the mediocre execution of a basic technique and a stunning demonstration of defensive skill. The flawless transmission of poomsae dramatically reflects this belief. While a great majority of modern forms have been exhaustively cataloged both in print and on the Web, many of the traditional poomsae dating back centuries are left to the mercy of memorization. Here is where the golden relationship between master and disciple clearly displays its value. A legitimate grandmaster with roots firmly planted in decades of Korean martial arts practice, who has doubtlessly performed advanced poomsae hundreds if not thousands of times, has the capacity to correct even the most minute detail within a given pattern. Left unattended, however, the practitioner may innocently promulgate error while infecting others, ultimately causing the execution of the poomsae, over time, to stray further and further from the core of its original intent. Grandmasters with an eye for the more traditional components of the taekwondo curriculum are also more likely to focus on authentic training in one-step sparring, self-defense techniques, meditation, and Ki development exercises as well.

Moreover, accumulated wisdom is generally a function of age. While there exists many youthful, talented grandmasters, acquired skill of this nature is generally attributed to those of advanced years. Time has a tendency of tempering their outlook on a discipline such as taekwondo making the grandmaster, in many cases, a teacher who is demanding yet compassionate, high in expectations yet forgiving of frailty. He or she is a wealth of knowledge, an advisor at times imparting thoughtful counsel and, as is the case with our grandmaster, a single, unifying symbol of a global organization. Physically, even those of senior rank, years older than their students, can inspire and elicit respect through the execution of basic technique performed effortlessly.

Accepting the leadership of a grandmaster removes the potential of being hindered by a provincial worldview of taekwondo. For the master instructor of a dojang not located in a large metropolitan area, interaction with colleagues can be minimal at best. Therefore, grandmasters with ties to others in the taekwondo community have the ability of introducing loyal students to peers of equal seniority and interests, opening the door to new relationships and unforeseen possibilities. Often a confederation of master instructors under the umbrella of a noted grandmaster can lead to mutual training experiences, seminars, association tournaments, and even trips to Korea—the homeland of taekwondo.

But at the end of the day, it is important to remember that the grandmaster is still only a human being commensurate with all the shortcomings that humble station entails. Students often mistakenly elevate the grandmaster to messianic proportions leaving themselves open to the dual specters of disappointment and disillusionment should their mentor's failings, for whatever reason, become evident. Therefore, just as the grandmaster showers his or her charges with compassion, so too must students exhibit genuine, unfailing understanding toward their senior.

Unquestionably, the mistaken assumption can be made that a master instructor's rate of maturity may be hindered by the influence of a seemingly oppressive grandmaster. Yet in reality, the master instructor who approaches the martial arts with humility will flourish in the shadow of a grandmaster whose sincere intent is to promote the traditions of taekwondo through the inculcation of wisdom, compassion, and technical excellence. I have personally witnessed this process through my own affiliation with my mentor, Grandmaster Richard Chun. Many hours have been shaved off my determined search for knowledge through his constant, unbiased guidance. But a single light can illuminate only the immediate area surrounding it no matter how bright. Fortunately, Grandmaster Chun and others like him have seen fit to transmit their hard-earned martial arts and life lessons to those worthy of their virtues. These individuals, some of whom we shall meet in the following section, are repositories of knowledge and represent the future of traditional taekwondo.

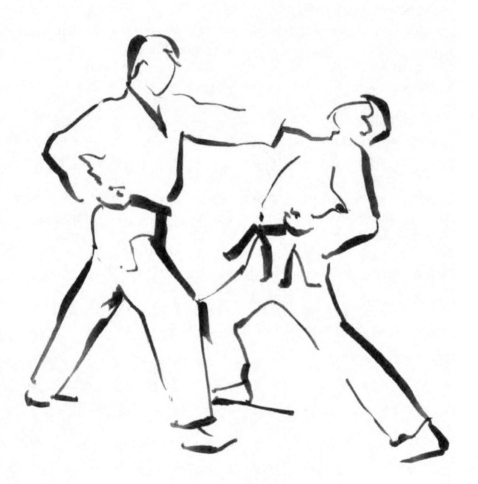

Part Five

My Students and Colleagues

The Dojang—A Safe Haven

On September 11, 2001, I was employed in New York City at a job that I would soon vacate in favor of teaching martial arts professionally. On that tragic but stunningly brilliant morning, I stood on the corner of Fifth Avenue and Nineteenth Street watching the destruction of the World Trade Center unfold before my very eyes.

Seconds after seeing the second plane slam into the South Tower, realizing full well that this was an assault on our country equal only in magnitude to the infamous attack on Pearl Harbor, I quickly made the decision to leave the city to seek the safety of my home and family sixty miles away.

Convincing a business associate that it would be best to flee the ensuing confusion, we shot up the FDR Drive in his car, listening as an incredulous radio personality announced the attack on the Pentagon, the crash of an airliner in Pennsylvania, and ultimately, the collapse of the Twin Towers. Anyone locally who bore witness to the rapidly unfolding disaster will appreciate the shock we both felt.

Almost three hours later, after plucking my children from the chaos of a terrified classroom and attempting to calm my wife upon our return home, I sat in my study fielding telephone call after telephone call inquiring as to my safety. Most were communications with friends and relatives, yet a significant amount of the calls originated from frightened and disoriented students. Was I safe? Is our taekwondo school open? Would classes be held today as scheduled? Answering in the affirmative to all three questions, I drove to the dojang with one thought in mind: as a martial artist and school owner who realized there was little any of us could personally do at this point, it was my mission to provide a sense of security and shelter for my anxious students. While people were flocking in droves to homes, social centers, and churches in every corner of the county, our students, who sought tranquility in taekwondo, were resolutely making their way to a place familiar to them, a place that offered a sense of community and collective comfort from the staggering events of the day.

I will never forget the mood in the dojang that evening. Yet I was not surprised given the literal translation of dojang—a place to study *The Way*. The tragedy brought our martial arts family together as a unit. Defined by our doboks, belts, and the rituals of our art, we began to train. Slowly the spirit of taekwondo took hold until—at least for a few hours—we enjoyed a respite from a world on the threshold of our community gone haywire. What was it about this physical space that worked its magic on us? What profound distraction could possibly supplant the mind-numbing sensations that roared through our brains like a hurricane, resonating in our bones?

It is not unusual for taekwondoists to feel a sense of comfort when they step into the dojang, a familiarity that adds consistency to an often hectic life. This is especially true when business or family matters result in a short-term absence. Returning, the practitioner crosses a spiritual boundary onto the training floor in the wake of the required bow of respect, glances in the mirror, and seeing his or her reflection is reminded of the nobility and perseverance associated with a diligent study of the traditional martial arts.

Furthermore, it is here in the dojang that a mutual respect is forged between those with a common goal, replacing the daily tug-of-war found in the workplace, schoolyard, or playing field. There is a giver and receiver of technique that alternates between individuals. In an extraordinary display of self-control, practitioners of all ages and both genders lend their bodies to one another in an effort to achieve personal excellence through the practice of an ancient and evolving art. In the ebb and flow of self-defense, one strikes, another blocks; one sweeps, another yields. It is this strange dance that promotes courtesy, focus, and reverence for tradition in the martial artist. Only in the safety of the dojang can these skills be fostered since it is understood what happens here remains here.

Moreover, a traditional dojang is built for utility and veneration of the art. Our national flag and that of the Republic of Korea adorn the wall. Sometimes, a scroll composed of rice paper scripted with calligraphy decorates an honored space, its flowing brush strokes representing a principle or ideal unique to the martial arts. Too, it is not a place devoid of color; often the training floor is covered with the bright array of a puzzle mat, radiating a pattern of contrasting hues. Aside from being a feast for the eyes, its functionality serves to protect the practitioner from the throws and sweeps found in traditional taekwondo. If mirrors are present, they are constantly wiped clear of smudges and fingerprints since the cleanliness of the dojang and all that it contains is a direct reflection of the technical precision expected from the students who fill it. Kicking targets, like a column of

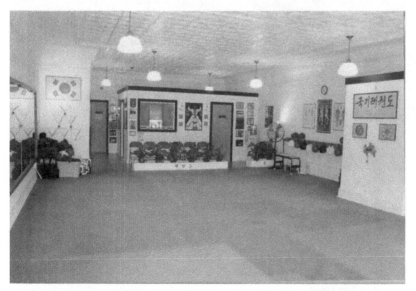

The training hall of the Chosun Taekwondo Academy.

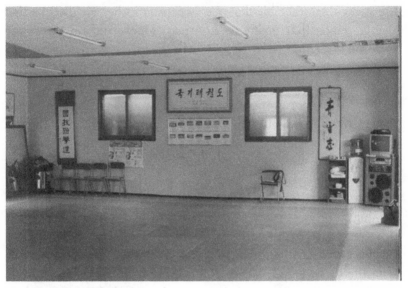

The dojang of Grandmaster Gyoo Hyun Lee in Yangsu-ri, South Korea.

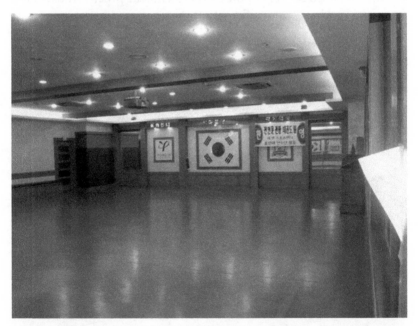

The Yong-In University dojang located in a suburb of Seoul, South Korea.

soldiers, hang on hooks in rows so neat a drill sergeant would approve. Although authentic taekwondo is defined as a weapon-less art, some schools cross-train in other Korean martial arts. If *kumdo* (The Way of the Sword) is a featured, secondary discipline, *jook do*, or bamboo swords, are to be found within quick reach. Likewise, *bong*, or fighting staff training, can be added to promote upper body strength and coordination and to act as a supplementary tool suited for self-defense.

The dojang is also a place for meditation and Ki develop-ment. This perhaps was the single most cleansing component of the traditional taekwondo core curriculum that satisfied our need for clarity on that infamous day. As we sat, hands resting in our laps describing an ancient mudra or hand gesture, eyes closed, feeling the smooth exchange of breath push away distraction, our minds soothed and a welcome calm began to pervade the room.

And so on that sunny September afternoon—a day that through the mercy of the mind is, for many of us, beginning to seem so distant yet will never be forgotten—all these elements conspired to provide a shell of serenity for those within. The sur-rounding four walls, floor, and ceiling, that without their custom-ary ornamentation could be construed as a mere room, combined to create a space to breathe and to organize emotion as we at-tempted to make sense of it all. For this is no ordinary living space; it is an environment filled with a courage commensurate with the rich tradition of the Korean martial arts. It is a dojang, a safe haven, a place to study *The Way*.

The Tradition of Training While Traveling

Dojangs can be found in the most unusual places. Today, for the most part, they are located in structures of brick, wood, glass, and steel. Yet this was not always the case. Decades ago, they were found in railway stations and on rooftops.[43] In centuries past, dojangs were situated behind temple walls and on training fields beneath the sun and stars. In many cases these physical spaces were filled with the yells of clerics adept in some form of defensive discipline. Moreover, it was not uncommon for warrior monks bearing martial arts skills to leave their temple dojangs and travel the countryside spreading technique and philosophical beliefs. One such monk was the Zen patriarch, Bodhidharma. The third son of a Brahman King, Bodhidharma left his native India in A.D. 526 and journeyed throughout China for many years until settling at the famed Shaolin Temple located in Hunan Province. There, according to legend, he transmitted his style of formal exercise, establishing the foundation for what would eventually become the various forms of Chinese martial arts.

Traveling Buddhist and Taoist monks in general benefited greatly from martial arts training in that it provided a means of unarmed self-defense against wild animals and roving bandits bent on robbing them of priceless religious icons and other valuables. Furthermore, we can imagine that members, most likely of the same sect, would compare or share techniques when coming together for various functions in the ancient monasteries located high in the mountainous regions of Asia.

Even though relatively few of us in the global martial arts community today are practicing clerics, there is no reason that we cannot take advantage of this tradition of training in distant dojangs while traveling regardless of whether our primary mission revolves around business or pleasure. In fact, paying a visit to a local dojang while far from home not only offers an opportunity to forge lasting friendships and enhance our overall knowledge of the martial arts, but in all likelihood will serve to remind us that the martial artist's basic desire to improve life through diligent training is universal. However, as with any worthy endeavor associated with the martial arts, there are rules relating to decorum that should be followed.

First and foremost, you should notify your instructor of your intentions. Often he or she may be familiar with the schools in a given area and not only make recommendations on where to train, but call ahead, paving the way for your visit. For various reasons, this practice should always be adhered to whether it is you or your instructor initiating the call. For instance, some insurance policies may preclude anyone but members from training at a certain facility. Or a particular school may teach a form of martial art totally unfamiliar to you. There is also the remote possibility that the doors of a school will be closed to non-members altogether. In my travels, I have found this last scenario to be the least likely. In fact, the courtesy, respect, and bonds we share as martial artists have been evident in every location I have had the honor of visiting.

In today's Internet world, it is easier than ever to seek out potential schools in which to train while traveling. Local businesses are usually listed on a city's Chamber of Commerce Web site or you can query the online Yellow Pages. For a more valuable training experience, try to select a school that features a style similar to the one you currently train in unless you are looking to sample something different. Remember to bring along a memento from your school such as a patch or tee shirt to give as a gift and always offer to pay for your training. Most schools will refuse payment for a single class but may request tuition if you intend to return for multiple sessions. Either way, the experience is well worth it.

During my travels I have experienced warm welcomes at dojangs in diverse locations ranging from Los Angeles to Atlanta, and from Amherst, Massachusetts, to Seoul, South Korea. Once, while on vacation in Cape Hatteras, North Carolina, I found the only dojang on the Outer Banks and trained vigorously for three consecutive evenings. On another occasion, I took advantage of an opportunity to train in California at a school affiliated with a dojang I had been training at in New York City. This worked out well since the routine, basic drills, and forms were identical to those I was familiar with.

But, aside from my training in Korea, perhaps one of my more memorable training experiences while traveling took place at the Kin-Tora Judo Club, a family-owned *dojo* located in Buffalo, New York. I had been searching the Web for a taekwondo dojang, but finding none I decided to visit a school that offered a variety of martial arts. While taekwondo was available, it was the aikido and judo classes that were scheduled the evening I arrived. Because I had previously requested permission to train, my appearance did not come as a surprise to the instructors. I was welcomed at the front desk, fitted with a judo *gi*, or heavy woven uniform, and not my standard V-neck taekwondo dobok, and invited to join the other practitioners already on the mat. What followed was an hour-long training session that mirrored the true essence of the martial arts. While I had never trained in judo prior to that evening, I was treated with patience and respect by all the students present. The highly capable instructor worked with me personally until I was gifted with five techniques that I am continuously working to perfect. Following the vigorous workout I was invited to join the owners, along with the other students, for refreshments and a stimulating discussion regarding their exciting martial art.

While I do not think that I possess the makings of an exemplary *judoka*, I hope the rewarding experiences I have described illustrate the value of training while traveling. Practitioners are exposed to different methods of training, new faces, and a fresh environment. But, perhaps most importantly, we experience the patience, honor, and courtesy inherent in the martial arts. Consequently, next time you find yourself packing for an excursion don't forget to include your dobok and belt.

A Woman's Touch

Not long ago, a middle-aged mother came to visit my school with her three adolescent daughters in tow. She proceeded to tell me a story that I have often heard before. It seemed that as a girl she had always dreamed of studying the martial arts, but was forbidden by parents who felt that it was inappropriate for a young lady to entertain such unorthodox notions. Finally, after all these years, she wanted to correct this misfortune and, committing to a program geared toward families, allow her children to share in her dream. Now, for these women, taekwondo is like a gift to be opened every day.[44]

Aside from their male counterparts, women of all ages find the practice of traditional taekwondo to be a highly rewarding experience. In truth more than half of our school's student population is female, and I am convinced that this ratio holds true in most dojangs across the nation. Yet for many years, during the genesis of the martial arts in America, it was unusual for a woman to train in taekwondo. "Dungeon dojangs" situated in cellars and back alleys, or in gyms exclusively for men, did little to provide even the most basic of training environments for the female practitioner and were often unsafe for either gender. Couple this with the fact that it was only within the past few decades that women began to penetrate the glass ceiling of martial arts in Korea and an inequitable social history slowly begins to materialize. Fortunately, this pattern was destined to be broken by the vanguard of women's rights that swept through Western culture, particularly in America, during the late twentieth century.

Today, there is little doubt that female practitioners benefit greatly from a sincere study of traditional taekwondo. Serenity of mind through meditation, confidence instilled by drilling in self-defense, physical fitness gained through vigorous training methods, all create an individual who is greater than the sum of her parts. This synergy can be seen as a vehicle for the empowerment of women in dojangs across the nation and, now, the world.

Moreover, it is not women who exclusively benefit from their participation in taekwondo, but the art of taekwondo itself that gains from a woman's touch. Aside from developing into sturdy martial artists, worthy competitors, and role models to all students, programs at many schools profit from the compassion and patience female instructors afford their eager pupils. Many, being mothers themselves, have a unique understanding of how to approach excitable youngsters attending children's classes that to some may prove problematic. Likewise, as is the case in our school, women instructors provide valuable insight when it comes to the composition of techniques that form women's self-defense courses. These highly capable teachers, more than anyone, appreciate the threats posed by a potential male predator and can interface with their peers in a serious and meaningful manner. Having practiced taekwondo skills against their male counterparts, female martial artists can realistically impart the importance of speed, balance, and the element of surprise in conjunction with the will to execute an effective defensive strategy. Whereas men mostly rely on strength, a woman must often rely on vital strategies in order to extricate herself safely from an altercation and who better to impart this knowledge than a member of the same gender.

Adding yet another dimension to their practice, rather than perceiving taekwondo as a pure form of self-defense, women, as well as men, can enjoy the discipline simply for the *art* of it. Keeping in mind that the traditional martial art of Korea is as much an avenue for expressing physical motion in the spatial plane as it is a valid system of self-defense, we can appreciate how spiritually uplifting the execution of precise technique can be. In fact, Grandmaster Sang Kyu Shim in his inspiring volume, *The Making of a Martial Artist*, likens the taekwondoist more to a dancer than a boxer, based on the agility and grace required by the art.

Lastly, and perhaps most importantly, resolutely stepping across the threshold of the dojang door and committing to a regimen of disciplined training categorically states that the female student refuses to assume the role of a potential victim—not simply to the threat of bodily harm but to the false notion that there is relatively little she can do to significantly alter her place in a society that has long discriminated against her gender. A reflection of this concept can been drawn from an article in the *Wall Street Journal* pointing out that employers are more likely to hire an individual who has practiced a martial art over other candidates due to the commitment, integrity, and self-control intrinsic to that pursuit. These attributes clearly bolster the worldview of any practitioner, but imagine what this perspective can do for individuals of either gender who have become accustomed to living under the shadow of psychological repression no matter how benign or unintentional?

It is useful to recall that taekwondo was originally created as a method of self-defense for soldiers on the field of battle. Moreover, it was proven effective during combat in the jungles of Vietnam and the Korean Conflict, the bloody civil war between citizens of the same nation. Is it any wonder then why women—who from time immemorial have been convinced of their physical inferiority when compared to their male counterparts—choose to embrace a legitimate, traditional Asian martial art that offers empowerment and a break with the conventional model of women as defenseless individuals?

Still, there are men who view the significant inroads women have made in taekwondo as a detriment to the male testosterone-laden workout. Recently, I bumped into an instructor who chose to leave his school due to an irreconcilable disagreement with the master instructor. A few weeks prior, he had approached me to request membership in our school. However, based on his somewhat dubious reputation, I refused. Upon meeting him again, I inquired as to how he was doing and if he were currently teaching. "I left taekwondo," he said with an air of triumph. "I'm practicing a real martial art now." He then went on to assert that taekwondo has evolved into nothing more than a woman's social club at most dojangs and how the curricula at these institutes were unfairly weighted toward that gender. Instead, he sought out a school where people "break bones and hurt each other—the real thing," he growled. Feeling vindicated about my decision not to accept this man as a student, I returned to my dojang where a midday adult class was about to begin. As I looked out over the group dominated by my female students, I felt a sense of pride in their acquired power, skillful precision, and newly-found confidence. Watching them perform poomsae and spar, executing well-placed jumping back and spinning hook kicks within inches of their partners' vital points, I could not help but think how my cynical instructor friend would feel if he came in full contact with any one of these techniques. Perhaps he would change his outlook of taekwondo after experiencing a woman's touch of this nature!

Yet the consequence associated with an effective defensive technique is no joking matter. Full contact to the body by an intentional, determined defensive strike or kick, without a doubt, is certain to result in disaster. This is an issue, as we shall see, that should be considered and appreciated by martial artists of all levels and styles.

The Reality of Consequence

One cold, rainy February evening, my wife and I went to see the film *Million Dollar Baby* featuring Clint Eastwood and Hilary Swank. For those unfamiliar with the story line, Swank plays the role of a young woman obsessed with becoming a world champion boxer under the tutelage of her coach, a hardened trainer portrayed by Eastwood, who is pursued by the ghosts of his past. Regardless of the fact that it is a stunning piece of cinematic craftsmanship worthy of its Oscar win, I left feeling depressed and hopeful at the same time: depressed due to the film's tragic ending and hopeful because of the realistic manner, fraught with brutal consequences, in which the fight sequences were graphically depicted.

The movie progresses with Swank learning the ropes from Eastwood and, subsequently, competing in a series of ever more challenging contests. The fight scenes are well choreographed leaving the viewers on the edge of their seats. Moreover, as the stakes rise, the bouts become more vicious with a plethora of devastating punches leaving their gruesome marks. At one point the fighter receives a strike that results in a broken nose with nothing of the blood and gore left to the imagination. In another segment a hook punch leaves an eye bleeding and swollen shut. Lastly, through a demonstration of extremely poor sportsmanship, the actress is left incapacitated for life. Oddly enough, I found these scenes hopeful in the sense that exposing the disturbing consequences of technique in full color on the big screen should give pause to practitioners and laypeople alike who falsely think that little or no real injury will result from the intentional use of martial arts skills. Yet it is not difficult to see why most people might be deceived into thinking otherwise.

Too often today, young people as well as adults are engaged with video games and watch programs that glorify the martial arts through violent, yet unrealistic, scenes of brutality. I am hard-pressed to believe that an adversary, despite the provocation, would quickly lift himself off the ground following a well-aimed spinning hook kick to the head. The subsequent result of an injury inflicted in this manner is seldom highlighted since it would not play well at the box office. Multiple punches punctuated by endless kicks, more often than not, do not even break the skin according to Hollywood. What this does in essence is remove the all-important ingredient of *consequence* from a highly lethal equation. Not that audiences, especially youngsters, necessarily need to see the tragedy beyond the drama for added entertainment, but there comes a point when the Um should be balanced by the Yang if the martial artist and general public are to fully appreciate the sustained result of an accurately placed martial arts technique.

In my experience, various occasions come to mind when I consider the ultimate effect of an unprotected, full contact strike to another human being. For instance, one of my first instructors, in the heat of his 4th dan examination, was performing a self-defense parody against four supposed adversaries attacking with knife, punch, gun, and club, advancing from different directions. As the student positioned across from the attacker with the knife, I was horrified to hear the sickening crack of bone coming in contact with bone. Accidentally, the instructor had grazed the head of his student with a spinning hook kick, knocking out his contact lenses in the process. We watched as a large, purple contusion erupted from the student's forehead as he staggered to the ground. Although he could not continue as a participant in the event, he fortunately did not sustain any permanent injury.

Likewise, in another incident, I was the culprit exhibiting poor self-control. I felt genuine feelings of remorse during a sparring match when I unintentionally split open the forehead of my partner with a downward back fist. He stood there, blood dripping into his eyes, deciding whether to strike back in anger or let the situation pass without vengeance. Fortunately for us both, he chose the latter, more intelligent option.

And then, of course, all of us share stories of intentional kicks finding their targets in tournament competition, some resulting in nothing more than a scratch and others ending in complications that eventually change the way the sport aspect of taekwondo is administered.

At the risk of contradicting myself, I am the first to remind my students when an inadvertent strike slips through during a particularly vigorous training session that "this ain't art class!" However, I am also the one to teach youngsters and adults alike that pain and suffering due to intentionally inflicted injury does not stop with the recipient; it continues to blossom outward like ripples on a pond affecting not only the victim, but also the attacker who now is in possible difficulty with the law, coupled with the loved ones of the injured and attacker who must now cope with the misfortune. In this example, I am attempting to instill the ensuing penalty of intended injury beyond the physical manifestations by reinforcing the extended cost—something the movies, computer games, and television seem to have largely ignored.

Of course, all of the above presupposes that in the dojang we are teaching authentic self-defense techniques and not merely sport. Clearly, good sportsmanship would include an ingredient of self-control coupled with the understanding that our intention in the ring is not to disable or subdue an attacker until the appropriate authorities arrive, but to dominate in a match of combat skill where there is a clear winner and loser. With this in mind, strikes to the back and lower portion of the body are forbidden, greatly reducing the risk of severe injury. Likewise, there are rules that limit the use of sweeps, arm locks, and throws. These regulations, although indispensable in a sportive environment, result in creating an artificial atmosphere where injury, as it should be, is discouraged, thus innocently exacerbating the deficiency of consequence—not so in effective self-defense training as it relates to traditional taekwondo. When practicing to incapacitate or subdue the instigator of an unprovoked attack, all rules are abandoned on both sides and the martial artist needs to respect the damage and legal liability the business end of a strike or kick can generate regardless of how it is depicted in the media.

The reality is that we are training in an authentic martial art and must accept the fact that the potential clearly exists to injure and be injured. Therefore, when faced with unavoidable life-threatening danger it is wise to recall an axiom shared by many in the law enforcement and martial arts communities regardless of the consequences: "It is better to be judged by twelve than to be carried by six."

Recognition

Just as in the case of *Million Dollar Baby*, recognition of a student's hard work by his instructor can literally mean the difference between years of prolonged, enthusiastic training and the distressing decision, based on discouragement, to prematurely halt practice. Whether black belt or novice, students seem to reach a tipping point during their training where the slightest hint of encouragement through acknowledgement can sway their outlook significantly. I can still recall the feeling as if it were yesterday, of winning "Student of the Month" following the reading of my essay at a promotion test many years ago. Being recognized by my instructors and peers filled me with delight and encouraged me to train even harder. Since then there have been many occasions where I have received honors and each time the wonder of the moment never leaves me. More than anything, these experiences have taught me the importance of recognizing others. Being recognized for achievement is a joy indifferent to age. Adults and adolescents alike benefit greatly from knowing their efforts are readily apparent to others. Yet for the martial artist, recognition is not steeped in arrogance, but in the quiet confidence gained through the enthusiastic support of his peers.

The most basic form of recognition in the martial arts is the measurable goal of earning a belt. Qualifying for the next gup, or grade, involves months of strenuous practice whereas progressing to subsequent dan, or degree status, is measured in years. When the day arrives and the student is awarded the new belt or receives an additional stripe, the satisfaction he exudes is almost palpable. Mix this with the possibility of being recognized for advanced skill and determination through awards, ceremonies, and competitions, and a recipe for imbuing self-esteem in students of all ages quickly becomes apparent.

But material symbols, while important, often pale at sincere words of encouragement and recognition from a senior student or instructor. Realizing that the practice of traditional taekwondo is not merely a forum for social interaction or an arena for mutual admiration and that positive recognition is frequently balanced by constructive criticism, it would be wise for instructors to remember the extraordinary influence words wield.

Names without the familiar experience of their direct attachment to faces and actions are a somewhat hollow association. Nonetheless, I feel it is important to recognize several colleagues who personify sturdy links in the great chain of martial arts knowledge. Their tireless efforts have indeed contributed greatly to the promotion of traditional taekwondo. Some have crossed oceans with me, to Korea, in the pursuit of core technique. Others have taught without financial gain to enrich the lives of their juniors. Still more, in the early years of life, are developing a singular focus and commitment to the art of taekwondo that is unheard of in today's frenetic society. Most are master instructors, instructors, assistant instructors, and leadership team members of the Chosun Taekwondo Academy, without whom our school would be a poorer place. Others are colleagues I have come in contact with over the course of my training, colleagues that have enriched my practice all the more. Naturally, it is to my teacher and mentor that I must first pay homage.

Grandmaster Richard Chun

What began as a means of protecting himself from the ruffians of post-war Korea evolved into a career spanning over half a century for Grandmaster Richard Chun—a man who has dedicated his life to promoting the art of taekwondo. He exemplifies the true spirit of the martial arts by virtue of the many trials and tribulations he was forced to overcome at an early age. Today, he oversees a vast ocean of loyal students who have been inspired by his teachings. In the late 1980s, Richard Chun received his 9th dan Kukkiwon black belt certification, establishing him as one of the highest-ranking International Master Instructors in the United States today.

At age eleven, Richard Chun began his formal martial arts education at the famed Moo Duk Kwan under the direction of

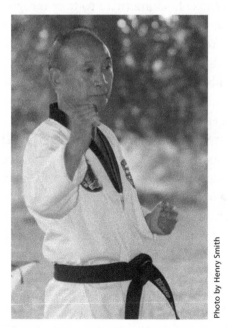

Photo by Henry Smith

Grandmaster Richard Chun, 9th dan black belt and president of the United States Taekwondo Association.

two highly respected teachers, Master Ki Whang Kim and Master Chong Soo Hong. By fourteen, having excelled in his training, he received his 1st dan black belt. Yet even now memories of his youth must, at times, be difficult. On June 25, 1950, North Korea invaded South Korea resulting in the outbreak of civil war. His father closed his medical practice and moved to the port city of Inchon in an effort to protect his family from the onslaught of Communist forces. During the cold winter of 1951, three families, including Grandmaster Chun's, fled south to Cheju Island in a small wooden boat, taking three weeks to complete the journey. Upon reaching his destination, fears of continuing his taekwondo training without the supervision of his master instructor flooded his mind. Attending high school at a rustic facility specifically designated for refugees, Richard Chun continued practicing taekwondo alone on the high mountain peaks of Mount Hallasan that overlooks the island. More than once his sense of justice and indomitable spirit were put to the test as the inhabitants of Cheju Island abused those flocking there to take refuge from the war.

In 1954, at age nineteen, he returned to Seoul. Once there, he enrolled in Yonsei University and graduated in 1957. While at the university, he continued his training, served as captain of the taekwondo club, and participated in several competitions. After graduating, Richard Chun worked for Air France in the position of sales manager for five years. Entering the United States in 1962 as a foreign student, he lived in Washington, D.C. and began studying for his Master's Degree in Business and Marketing at George Washington University. Five months later, he decided on a move that would change the complexion of taekwondo in the United States forever.

Twenty-eight years old and a newcomer to New York City, Grandmaster Chun began teaching taekwondo at a large health club in midtown Manhattan. Then, in 1964, with the assistance of past WTF president Dr. Un Yong Kim, he officially established the Richard Chun Taekwondo Center, a school that has cultivated champions such as Joe Hayes and catered to movie stars and sports figures alike.

While establishing a martial arts school and recruiting new students is often a difficult endeavor, an interesting turn of events landed the burgeoning school owner fifteen new students in one fell swoop. One evening, while enjoying a cocktail in a Greenwich Village tavern, six thugs approached the young martial artist and his companion demanding that they give them money. The group left after receiving three dollars, but quickly returned for more. Told that none would be forthcoming, the situation turned violent. Acting in self-defense, Chun rendered two of the group unconscious using taekwondo skills while the remaining four dispersed. A *New York Post* reporter who happened to be passing by, took notice, which resulted in his writing an article in the paper the following day. After reading the article, likely candidates for taekwondo training began calling and the budding martial arts center began to grow. For decades, the Richard Chun Taekwondo Center remained a Mecca for practitioners locally and worldwide who sought out the teachings of the legendary grandmaster.[45]

Between working and teaching, Grandmaster Chun earned his master's degree at Long Island University. He eventually went on to obtain a Ph.D., becoming a professor of health and physical education at Hunter College in New York City.

In 1973, Grandmaster Chun was appointed head coach of the U.S. Taekwondo Team, leading them to a second-place victory in the first World Taekwondo Championships held in Seoul, South Korea.

Ralph Waldo Emerson once wrote that "an institution is the lengthened shadow of one man." This axiom is uniquely true of Richard Chun who, in 1980, went on to establish the USTA, an organization whose mission is to promote the ancient and evolving art of taekwondo. A non-profit, professional entity devoted to the development and progression of taekwondo both as a traditional martial art and a world sport, the USTA provides guidance in establishing national standards of practice, competition, testing, and accreditation for its members. It is an active member of the WTF, the prime force in the recognition of taekwondo as an Olympic sport by the IOC.

Grandmaster Richard Chun also played a major role in organizing taekwondo as an event in the 1988 Olympic Games and has served as Senior International Referee at subsequent championships and Olympic competitions. For his many achievements in promoting taekwondo within the borders of the United States, he received the Presidential Award from the president of Korea. In 1990, he was named Special Assistant to the president of the WTF. He has also received many citations over the years from the Moo Duk Kwan and the WTF. In 2008, Grandmaster Chun was appointed Overseas Special Advisor to the Kukkiwon.

As if these accomplishments were not sufficient enough to secure his place in the annals of taekwondo history, Grandmaster Chun shares his knowledge of taekwondo through the written word with five books to his credit, all of which have been translated into several foreign languages. These books remain a standard in the martial arts community and are used as reference guides by thousands of practitioners and schools worldwide.

The Masters of the USTA

Being accepted as a student by Grandmaster Chun was a high honor and a form of recognition beyond my wildest expectations as a color belt. I received my 2nd dan just after I became a member of the Richard Chun Taekwondo Center. With mixed emotions, I had recently left a school that disappointingly placed significant commercial gain over tradition. However, once I was exposed to the core curriculum and became acquainted with the instructors that taught at Grandmaster Chun's dojang, any doubt that may have existed in my mind quickly evaporated. My first few classes at the school were overseen by Master Samuel Mizrahi, Master Pablo Alejandro, and the late Master Thomas James. Later, I met and had the privilege of training under Master Fred Kouefati, Master Bill Canagaeta, Master Richard Conceicao, Master Geraldine Michalik, and Guinness Book world-record holder for breaking solid objects, Master Maurice Elmalem. These master instructors represented a brain trust unequaled within the confines of many schools. Each possessed unique skills and training methods based on the teachings of Grandmaster Chun. Many, at one time or another, directed branch schools. To this day, I continue to train with Grandmaster Chun, Master Mizrahi, and Master Alejandro. Their enthusiasm for traditional taekwondo is infectious, and I am constantly inspired by their technique and wisdom.

On several occasions in the past my students have accompanied Grandmaster Chun and me on training and cultural tours of Korea. Aside from appreciating the rich, native heritage of the Korean people, we were given an opportunity to train with some of the most noted instructors in the world. Included in this elite group of professionals were Grandmaster Gyoo Hyun Lee, Grandmaster Sang Hak Lee, Master Sang Bum Yoon, and Master Ryan An.

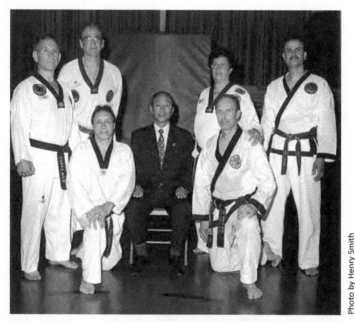

Photo by Henry Smith

USTA Master Instructors with Grandmaster Richard Chun: (standing left to right) Maurice Elmalem, Samuel Mizrahi, Amanda Haddock, Fred Kouefati; (seated) Grandmaster Richard Chun; (kneeling left to right) Pablo Alejandro, Doug Cook.

Grandmaster Gyoo Hyun Lee

Both in the media and in person, Grandmaster Gyoo Hyun Lee cuts a striking image; with a shock of white hair centered over the left eye, in concert with his drill sergeant demeanor, his presence is unmistakable. Although in his early sixties, he moves like a cat. His flexibility, enthusiasm, and strength are in direct proportion to his long years of dedication to the art of taekwondo. He is currently president of the World Taekwondo Instructor Academy and director of the Kukkiwon Taekwondo Training Center. From 1990 to 1998, his abilities earned him the position of Chairman, Training Subcommittee, Kukkiwon, and prior to that, from 1973 to 1982, he was head of the Kukkiwon Demonstration Team. Grandmaster Lee and his colleague, Master Kook Hyun Jung, have been chosen by the WTF and the Kukkiwon to model in a series of instructional DVDs aimed at standardizing the Taegeuk, and WTF Yudanja series poomsae. These training tools are

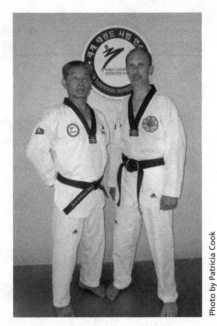

Photo by Patricia Cook

Grandmaster Gyoo Hyun Lee (left) with the author at the headquarters dojang of the World Taekwondo Instructor Academy in Yangsu-ri, South Korea.

intended to be used as a reference for referees, coaches, instructors, and competitors preparing to participate in WTF Poomsae World Championships.

Grandmaster Sang Hak Lee

I met Grandmaster Sang Hak Lee in 1999 during a training tour of Korea. He was responsible for teaching the Korean Army Ranger Corps and National Police Agency self-defense tactics and was head of a select team of martial artists sent to Vietnam to demonstrate the practicality of taekwondo. During our time together, Grandmaster Lee, a tall, trim man with a ruddy complexion, moved effortlessly through the various self-defense techniques with which he chose to gift us. He allowed his opponent's aggressive behavior to betray him through the blending and redirection of punches, kicks, and grabs, thus demonstrating the true defensive philosophy of traditional taekwondo. He did not speak much, choosing instead to perform each technique with the

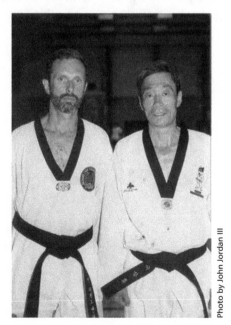

Photo by John Jordan III

Grandmaster Sang Hak Lee (right) with the author, following an intense class focusing on ho sin sool.

spirit we come to expect from an experienced Korean master. By the end of the afternoon, somewhat bruised and overwhelmed, we were given over twenty self-defense tactics to take home to America.

Master Sang Bum Yoon

Master Sang Bum Yoon is a cheerful, young martial artist when compared to many of his seasoned seniors. He speaks English fluently and is quick to smile. Aside from managing the taekwondo program at Yong-In University, he is a graduate of the Hwarang Educational Institute, a professional instructor, and acted as our liaison during the Chosun Taekwondo Academy 1999 Korea Training Camp. Each morning, in a small courtyard behind our hotel, with the sunrise warming our night-stiffened bodies, Master Yoon would lead us in what he referred to as "morning exercises." Typically, our group was directed to begin by forming a circle. Master Yoon would then execute a series of flexibility exercises similar to those we practiced back home and continued

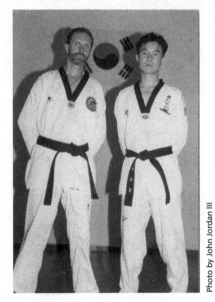

Photo by John Jordan III

Master Sang Bum Yoon (right) with the author at Kyung Won University in Seoul, South Korea.

with a set of drills emphasizing advanced footwork, or *baljitki*. Defense kicks, as he called them, were added to complete the stepping patterns and I remember thinking that we were being shown techniques uniquely Korean in nature, unlike any I had experienced previously. Several years later Master Yoon spent time at my home while visiting America. Each day, he would accompany me to the dojang and teach very difficult classes. He advised me to move into the space my school presently occupies saying that if we followed his advice, our school would prosper and grow.

Master Ryan An

In the past, Hoki Taekwondo (Little Tiger Taekwondo) occupied a large room at the Korean War Memorial Museum. That is where I originally met and trained with Master Ryan An. He, too, is a young master and has since moved his dojang to a new location in Seoul. A devoted family man, Master An possesses a deep love for taekwondo that is evident in his passionate approach to teaching. Strict and demanding, he requires total commitment

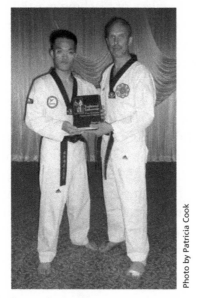

Photo by Patricia Cook

Master Ryan An (left) with the author, following a training session at Hoki Taekwondo in Seoul, South Korea.

from his students. Master An is a colleague of Grandmaster Gyoo Hyun Lee and is affiliated with the World Taekwondo Instructor Academy. He is also responsible for developing an exceptional demonstration team that regularly performs for visiting tourists.

The Teachers and Students of the Chosun Taekwondo Academy

Teaching traditional taekwondo professionally is a blessing that I give thanks for each and every day! Having the ability to pursue my passion while affecting the lives of others in a positive manner confirms to me all the more that I am fulfilling my destiny.

The Chosun Taekwondo Academy, while not the biggest dojang in our town, maintains a solid reputation for traditionalism and has been successfully operating for many years. However, without the commitment and loyalty of my students and instructors, none of this would be possible. Many of our senior instructors and assistants, including John Jordan III, Terri Testa, Richard Tamian, and Danielle Roche, have been with our school since its creation. Others, equally as competent, have more recently earned the privilege of teaching martial arts at Chosun. Included in this group are Cheryl Crouchen, Peter Brawley, Raoul Ratsep, Robert Adams, Christopher Songer, Elizabeth Quasius, James Vandenburg Jr., Terrie Wynne, and Brian Fitzsimmons. All, without exception, transmit traditional taekwondo philosophy, customs, and technique with compassion and a true understanding of the art. Yet, above all, it is essential to recognize our students and the youthful members of our Leadership Team for their dedication to the Chosun Taekwondo Academy and the art of taekwondo, for enthusiastically coming to class morning, noon, and night, for enduring the difficult training we demand, and for taking control of their lives through a diligent study of the traditional martial arts. It has been an honor to instruct my students and watch them grow.

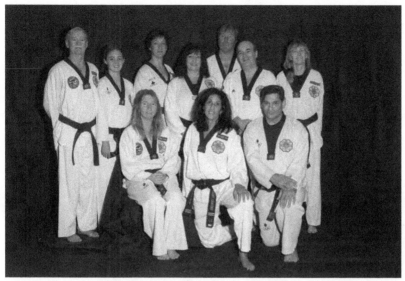

The Instructors of the Chosun Taekwondo Academy located in Warwick, New York; (standing from left to right) James Vandenburg Jr., Samantha Testa, Terrie Wynne, Patricia Lurye, Raoul Ratsep, Robert Adams, Danielle Roche; (seated and kneeling) Terri Testa, Cheryl Crouchen and Richard Tamian.

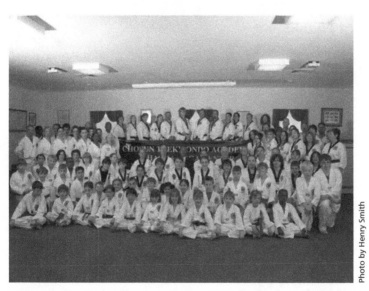

The Chosun Taekwondo Academy 10th anniversary promotion examination.

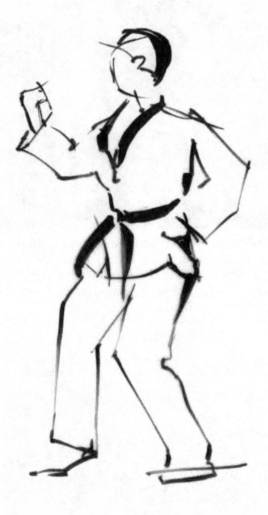

Part Six

Economics of
the Martial Arts

The Grand Mosaic

Maintaining a uniquely traditional martial arts academy as we have at Chosun requires a balance between the grand mosaic of physical skill that comprises taekwondo and commercial solvency. This equilibrium is repeatedly challenged by the sincere school owner's desire to preserve the often mystical Asian customs surrounding the martial arts and consistently putting food on the table. Consequently, the contemporary manager searches for methods to motivate students while providing them with authentic martial arts instruction in conjunction with a road to spiritual enhancement and physical fitness—never an easy chore. This dichotomy represents the economic decisions that need to be recognized when teaching martial arts today.

Understandably, master instructors I come in contact with share a common concern when enrollment in their school either stagnates or, at worst, declines. In response, program directors responsible for growth frequently turn to instruments such as financially obligatory, multi-year contracts in an effort to secure sustained membership. While this practice is understandable given the Western belief that money is the ultimate motivator, there remain other, less onerous methods available to promote student retention. These solutions, however, rely more on a comprehensive knowledge of the technical principles intrinsic to *traditional* taekwondo than they do on shrewd business practice. An article written some years ago by the late martial artist Jane Hallander entitled "Is Taekwondo a Sport or Self-Defense System?" hints at the inherent dangers associated with ignoring these preferences. The author suggests that locating a dojang still teaching traditional taekwondo will become increasingly difficult as time goes on. Moreover, finding an instructor sufficiently competent to transmit these unique skills to those worthy of its virtues will become even more difficult.

Clearly, due to its Olympic status, many schools currently focus primarily on the combat sport element of taekwondo, an aspect steadfastly developed through the efforts of the WTF. However, by highlighting the requirements for successful competition in the ring, many of the techniques and philosophical underpinnings associated with self-defense, including hand techniques, Ki development, and meditation, have been subjugated or forfeited altogether. These overlooked yet quintessential components of traditional taekwondo constitute a grand mosaic that must be presented in its entirety if the student is to receive a holistic education in this truly authentic martial discipline.

By now, we should be familiar with the pieces of the puzzle that formulate the richly diverse and efficient curriculum unique to traditional taekwondo. Certainly, development of the mind, body, and spirit must be addressed in accordance with the ability to defend against an unprovoked attack. Other vital elements identified earlier include training in one-, two-, and three-step sparring as well as ho sin sool practice. But perhaps the most significant inlay that completes the grand mosaic is the recognition of poomsae and how the formal exercises relate to the various styles of taekwondo. Whether they are the Palgwe or Taegeuk series fashioned by the WTF, or the twenty-four tul in the Chang-Han set created by ITF founder General Choi Hong Hi, formal exercises represent the essence of any classical martial art. In his 1975 book, *Moving Zen*, Shotokan practitioner C.W. Nicol described formal pattern practice as "a dynamic dance, a battle without bloodshed or vanquished." He further goes on to say that by performing poomsae, "we are somehow touching the warrior ancestry of all humanity" and that "of all the training in karate, none is more vigorous, demanding or exhilarating than the sincere performance of kata."[46] From this we can see that poomsae training, if approached in a traditional manner, cultivates self-defense skills, agility, focus, breath control, and, in most cases, strength coupled with Ki development.

Certainly, there is nothing wrong or sinister with combining healthy profits with a complete curriculum based on *traditional* taekwondo training. This formula is almost certain to keep schools financially solvent and accessible to those investing the patience to seek them out. Furthermore, an educational experience of this nature permits the student to advance in a progressive, orderly fashion challenging the mind, body, and spirit. Moreover, it is important not to give this art away, especially if it has been enhanced by constant practice on the part of the instructor. Yet, in order to successfully transmit traditional taekwondo skills in the manner described above, the practitioner must make the distinction between *teaching* martial arts and *practicing* martial arts.

Pursuing a Career in the Martial Arts

Many years ago, a good friend of mine related a story that I will never forget. An avid golfer, playing as many as four rounds a week, he decided to quit his job in the music business and open a pro shop selling golf-related equipment. He found the enterprise highly enjoyable and stimulating—at least for the first few months. Following this "honeymoon," it quickly became apparent that *selling* golf supplies was radically different from *playing* golf. In fact, given the reality that he was top man in a one-man venture, he rarely found the time to get out on the green at all. Eventually, the glamour of owning his own business, working days, nights, and on weekends, wore off and he found himself in a position that transformed his passion into an unpleasant chore.

Unhappily, this scenario happens all too often to the practicing martial artist as well. Young people, highly proficient in kicking, punching, and sparring, see an opportunity to parry their hard earned skills into a commercially viable profession. They arrange financing that is tenuous at best, search out an appropriate location in a strip mall, print up and distribute flyers, and open their doors hoping to attract enough students to pay the bills. After a few months of struggle, teaching day and night, recruiting students, collecting tuition, cleaning floors, toilet bowls, sinks, windows, and mirrors, they glumly realize that running a professional martial arts school is not the same as personal martial arts training.

Having said this, I would not trade what I do for anything in the world. It hasn't always been easy, but it has been enormously rewarding both professionally and spiritually. The reason for the success of our school is partially due to the fact that I never deluded myself into thinking that running a martial arts business was synonymous with *training* in taekwondo. The two, while certainly related, are exclusive to one another and must be viewed in that manner to insure continued success.

There are a number of elements that compound to create a working martial arts studio. Continuity is one. We offer classes from five-thirty in the morning till nine at night. If I or my instructors decided we didn't feel like getting up before sunrise one morning to teach, our students would quickly lose faith in our determination and commitment. Furthermore, not providing an authentic taekwondo curriculum based on a repeating, ever-evolving template of basic skills, forms, and self-defense can potentially confuse and frustrate students. I have heard horror stories of schools changing expectations on a weekly basis. Offering a program that practitioners can count on year in and year out screams of consistency and professionalism.

Another important component is a sincere knowledge of the martial art your school specializes in. In our case traditional taekwondo is what we teach. Our instructors are not only versed in the proper dynamics and purpose of the various kicks, blocks, and strikes that we seek to instill in our students, but are also knowledgeable regarding Korean history, terminology, and the rich philosophical underpinning that supports our martial way. This demonstrates to the student body that our staff truly desires to transmit a holistic version of taekwondo that enriches the mind, body, and spirit.

Nevertheless, all the academic and physical skill in the world will not come to the school owner's aid when the rent comes due. Aside from continuity and knowledge, business savvy is a must. Personally, I enjoyed a background in management and applied the acumen I gained over the decades to the operation of my school. Providing a clean, safe training environment, reaching out to the community with clear, concise marketing tools, maintaining accurate and up-to-date financial records, dealing with students in a balanced, professional manner, developing a reputation for paying vendors in a timely fashion are but a few of the practices that stimulate continued business. In this regard my experience enabled me to focus effectively on these essential requirements. I possessed knowledge in managing a physical plant, overseeing accounts payable and receivable, and dealing with human resources. However, for those wanting in commercial ability there are any number of martial arts management companies vying for business. These entities offer consultation, advertising tools, billing services, and a modicum of assistance in developing a curriculum. But it must be remembered that the transmission of traditional taekwondo from master to disciple is not only about dollars and cents as many of these companies would have you believe. In fact, some are so blatantly obvious about their thirst for monetary gain that it is profoundly disturbing to see. Clearly, we as martial arts professionals are responsible for the well being, both physically and spiritually, of our students. In my experience these noble souls do not attend dojangs across America to be sold false principles and products; they come to learn authentic, uncorrupted martial arts untainted by excessive personal gain— gain that is largely blind to the true virtues of taekwondo.

Unquestionably, when you assume the mantle of operating a traditional taekwondo institute you tacitly accept the fact that you walk a razor's edge between ethical instruction and commercial solvency. This is an exercise in balance, in the Um and Yang of the martial arts, that not all can accomplish. Falling victim to the lure of the almighty dollar is a temptation often hard to resist especially given the potential revenue generated operating a well-grounded school.

Furthermore, having long ago realized the important distinction between supporting a working martial arts school and increasing my personal skill in taekwondo, I make it a point to train with my grandmaster and his senior instructors at least once a week. This requires a four hour commute to and from the dojang, yet it is unjust to sit back and expect to motivate the students who rely on my abilities while my technique declines due to lack of personal training. Above all, taekwondo is an action philosophy and as such must be practiced diligently on a continuing basis for the instructor to remain proficient. Therefore, in the end, the business person in the equation must coexist with the martial artist in order to provide balance in the pursuit of success.

Aside from owning and operating a full-time dojang, there are other avenues a person can pursue in fostering an income through the martial arts. If you are so inclined, authoring books, articles, or columns, as I do, is an option. As martial artists, we appreciate the benefits of nurturing discipline. Writing requires a great deal of this virtue but it is, as is teaching, a spiritually rewarding proposition. There is a Taoist proverb that states: "Share your knowledge . . . it is a way to achieve immortality." By having others benefit from your acquired wisdom through the written word, you are providing a service that will reach across the years to those you would perhaps never meet—an achievement of profound worth. And then, of course, if you possess the physical attributes and skill of a Steven Segal or Cynthia Rothrock and have developed the necessary connections in Hollywood, you may be lucky enough to find gainful employment performing martial arts in the cinema or on television. Frankly, I don't think I need to be concerned with this option!

On reflection, whether you are a school owner, author, or movie star, perhaps the martial arts were never meant to be taught for monetary gain in the first place. Indeed, in years gone by it was not unusual for potential students to barter for lessons by offering the instructor household goods, food, or labor. But first they needed to convince the master that they were worthy of his teachings. Once accepted, actual technique was frequently prefaced by a seemingly nonsensical period of conditioning; the mind, body, and spirit needed to be hardened for the rigors ahead. There were no fancy uniforms, patches, belts, or membership contracts to motivate or bind a student to a school, just difficult and often painful training in a severe environment meted out by a demanding instructor. This model may have worked in feudal times, but would prove unrealistic from both a humanitarian and legal perspective in our modern social and fiscal environment. But it is a different wind that blows in Korea, a wind tinged with the scent of intensity and indomitable will. There, in the homeland of taekwondo, training methods and expectations by instructors radically exceed those we have become familiar with in the West. It is my belief that any potential school owner with commercial aspirations in mind should journey to the "Land of the Morning Calm" in order to gain a better understanding of the manner in which traditional taekwondo should be taught.

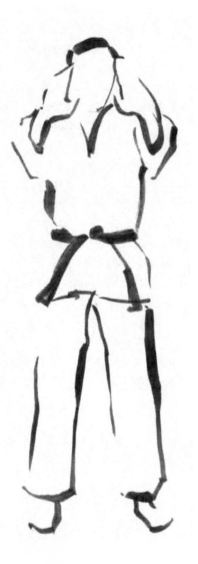

Part Seven

Visiting Korea: Land of the Morning Calm

Training in Korea: A Stressful Trip, But a Warm Welcome

Having traveled to Korea on several occasions, I feel strongly that we must experience the culture of this vibrant nation firsthand in order to fully understand the roots of taekwondo. In doing so, practitioners can make a geographical and historical connection with their physical training while sampling the unique heritage of the Korean people. Visiting the Kukkiwon, the various dojangs and universities, and meeting the many gifted masters and students of the art adds color and meaning to our practice that can be appreciated only by traveling to the homeland of taekwondo.

To date, I have acted as tour administrator for four excursions to Korea. The experience I have gained in arranging these journeys is worth passing on to those interested in doing the same. First, a bit of advice: planning and finally executing a trip of this nature can prove daunting, especially when traveling with a large group of students to various parts of the Korean countryside. The rewards, however, are great—unlike any the martial artist will discover locally. Preparations for making such a journey, while removing provincial boundaries from the mind, must be made carefully.

There are two possible routes you can take when planning this type of educational adventure. The first is to contact either a travel agency or martial arts organization in Korea that has prior experience in arranging group tours focusing on taekwondo.[47] I usually complete this phase of the excursion at least ten months in advance. This choice instantly eliminates a number of potential difficulties since any worthwhile package will include roundtrip airfare, lodging at quality hotels, dining at predetermined restaurants, training fees, admission to a variety of tourist attractions, and transportation via motor coach with an English-speaking guide. You can also attempt to make arrangements piecemeal by contacting dojangs, hotels, eating establishments, and transportation facilitators individually. This is tricky at best unless you or your master instructor has reliable contacts in-country. Very likely, there will be a language barrier to deal with in conjunction with a multiplicity of money transfers and contractual obligations. Frankly, I would recommend following the former strategy rather than the latter. Once the logistical hurdles have been cleared, all that remains is the anticipation you and your fellow travelers will share until the day of departure; and I can tell you firsthand . . . the emotion is palpable! One last suggestion before we depart on our journalistic tour to the "Land of the Morning Calm": clear your mind of any expectations or preconceived notions regarding your visit. Do not be concerned with what you will eat, where you will stay, or how hard you will train.[48] Cultivate a Zen mind and simply *be there* when you arrive.

In retrospect, I believe the most stressful part of a training and cultural tour to Korea is getting there in the first place.

Our long-awaited journey begins with a three-hour bus ride from upstate New York to Kennedy International Airport where twenty-five anxious students, including me, board an American Airlines DC-10 to Los Angeles. Sitting at the terminal for hours following check-in, we cannot wait to depart. The evening flight across the country is uneventful. I prepare my journals for the handwritten data that will fill them while my students play cards, unwind, and eventually sleep. We arrive in California five and half hours later only to find that Asiana flight 221 is being prepared for embarkation at the International Departure Terminal clear across the airport. Since our bags cannot be checked through due to security reasons, we must carry them ourselves for what seems like miles. My last trip to Korea taught me to pack light for mobility. Because I passed this lesson on to my students, the transfer is not as taxing as it could be. Two hours later,

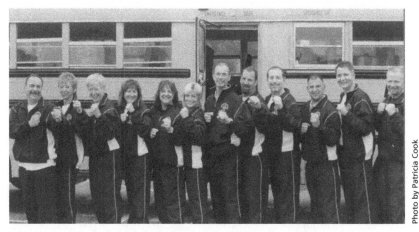

Photo by Patricia Cook

Chosun Taekwondo Academy students preparing to leave for the 2004 Korea Training & Cultural Tour.

3 A.M. Eastern Standard Time, we settle in and our huge Boeing 747-400 thunders down the runway bound for Seoul, South Korea. Having gotten our second wind, we realize that our journey has truly begun. The safety instructions announced by the flight crew are delivered in Korean and English over the communication system; magazines and newspapers are printed in hangul, the twenty-four character alphabet created in 1443 during the reign of King Sejong and still very much the pride of the Korean people today. Again, our anticipation begins to peak. During the long hours over the Pacific, we watch two movies, read, eat twice, and struggle to get some much needed rest. Sooner than hoped, the small coach seat I am buckled in seems to shrink around me. I look and notice my students, too, are beginning to fidget. It will be a long night.

Abruptly, I am awakened from a fitful sleep by lights blinking on throughout the cabin. I can smell the aroma of fresh coffee. The flight attendants announce that breakfast is being served and that we will be approaching the Korean peninsula shortly. Following our morning meal, I gaze out the window, straining my eyes to be the first to see our final destination. And then, suddenly, there it is, shrouded in mist, jagged mountain peaks lit by the first rays of sunrise . . . Korea: "Land of the Morning Calm."

Our pilot and crew guide the enormous silver bird in for an unusually soft landing and passengers applaud. We leave the main runway of Kimpo International Airport and taxi to a gateway at the International Arrivals Building. The oversized jet finally comes to a full stop and butterflies begin to invade my stomach. We have arrived. Being the administrator of this trip, I am genuinely hoping that everything progresses smoothly.

On this training and cultural tour we are fortunate beyond measure to be accompanied by martial arts pioneer Grandmaster Richard Chun, president of the USTA. Grandmaster Chun had left three days earlier to meet with colleagues from the WTF, the Kukkiwon, and the KTA in preparation for our visit. Clearly, doors that typically remain closed to Westerners open wide in Dr. Chun's presence. He is to meet us at the gate along with members of The Organizing Committee for Taekwondo Korea (TOCTK), our hosts for the next seven days.

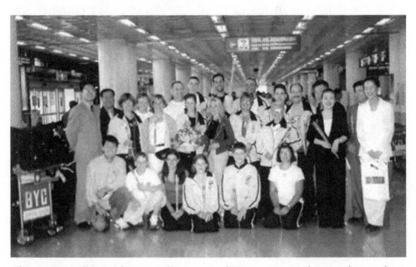

Chosun Taekwondo Academy students are welcomed as they arrive in Seoul for the 1999 Korea Training & Cultural Tour.

After clearing Republic of Korea customs, claiming our luggage, and exchanging our dollars for *won*, the ornate Korean currency, we enter the building's lobby and search the awaiting faces for our associates. It does not take long to pick them out. A large banner is unfurled bidding us welcome. There are women with flowers, and standing in the middle of it all is Grandmaster Chun, his smile as bright as the day around us. I can tell that he, like all of us, is very excited to be here.

Training in Korea: Kyung Won University

After connecting with Grandmaster Chun and our hosts from TOCTK at Kimpo International Airport, we are driven by motor coach to the Hotel TEMF. There, our weary group recuperates from the arduous journey through many time zones. Following a traditional Korean meal, we meet for an orientation session, receive uniforms from the TOCTK, and later in the evening, enjoy a festive ceremony attended by representatives from the WTF, the KTA, and the Kukkiwon. Many high ranking officials are present to demonstrate their respect for Grandmaster Chun. We return to our rooms relatively early since our training is to begin at sunrise the next day. I choose to reside in a traditional *ondol* room with a sleeping mat stretched out on the floor as would a native Korean while traveling throughout his or her country. It is good to sleep in a reclined position after spending so much time in a cramped airline seat. Next morning we awake, participate in morning exercises at the hotel offered by Master Sang Bum Yoon, take breakfast at a local restaurant, and board our motor coach for a short trip to the first destination on our itinerary.

Kyung Won University is located at 65 Bokjung-Dong in the Sujung-gu district of Seoul. Its sprawling campus contains all the modern facilities one would expect of a thriving academic institution. But, unlike its Western counterparts, Kyung Won offers a major in taekwondo. Potential students apply from all over the country in the hope of gaining admittance to what is perhaps one of the most intense martial arts training programs in the world.

On the top floor of a building situated in the center of the complex is the university's training hall. As we climb the circular flight of concrete steps leading to the entrance, I realize that over eight thousand miles and nearly two days' journey separate us from home and this much-anticipated moment in time. After changing into our doboks, we enter a training area measuring roughly fifty by one-hundred feet. Kicking targets, heavy bags, head gear, and chest protectors, or hogu, line the perimeter of the room. Shafts of natural light stream in through the tall windows that peak at the arched ceiling amplifying the contrasting colors of the orange and green puzzle mat. A banner beckoning us to embrace the "Dream of Taekwon" hangs above the entry way. We are called to attention in strict military fashion by Master Jang Ki Park, a professor of taekwondo at the university. Bows of respect are exchanged between the instructors, our group, the Kyung Won students, and members of the Syrian national taekwondo team, there, coincidently, to mutually participate in this advanced training program.

As a prelude to our practice we begin with a set of exercises intended to condition the muscles and heat the body's core. These consist of jumping jacks, sit-ups, push-ups, and static stretches followed by a series of relays. Mindful of building team spirit, we run, jump, evade, and crawl in six lines of ten students each, from one end of the dojang to the other.[49] Prepared now for an increase in intensity, the kicking drills begin in earnest. Kyung Won students sporting the university's logo on the back of their doboks stand at the head of each line holding a kicking target. One by one we execute round, hook, spinning hook, jumping round, turning back, and push kicks in an effort to enhance our technique. Blood-chilling kihops punctuate the strikes delivered by the Korean students. A 3rd dan at the time, I am intimidated by the high level of proficiency exhibited by these outstanding martial artists. The Kyung Won student wielding a kicking paddle at the head of our line notices my apprehension and offers an

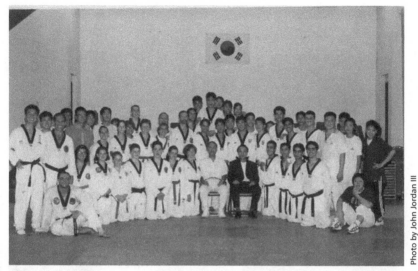

Photo by John Jordan III

Students of the Chosun Taekwondo Academy, Kyung Won University Taekwondo Team and the Syrian National Team following a training session at Kyung Won University.

encouraging smile. I am intent on performing flawlessly my next time up and when I correctly complete the technique, the student nods approvingly.

An hour later we begin to practice poomsae. Since the university adheres to the rules and regulations of the WTF, color belts practice the Taegeuk series while the various dan grade black belts perform Koryo, Keumgang, Taebaek, Pyongwon, and Sipjin according to rank.

Thoroughly exhausted after three hours of solid training, we break for lunch. Our hosts treat us to bulgogi—marinated beef over rice, complemented by kimchi, the ubiquitous pickled cabbage served with every meal. Following this delicious repast, we attempt to regain our strength by lounging in a shady, open-air pavilion beneath the ginkgo trees that line the campus.

At the resumption of our training, Master Park, presumably sensing the effect the hot afternoon is having on his students, begins with a remarkable method of *dynamic* meditation.[50] Seated

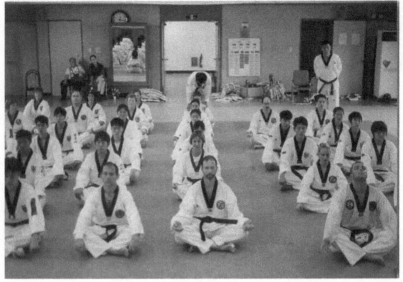

Ki development exercises lead by Master Jang Ki Park (rear).

in a half-lotus position, we perform a deep breathing exercise conjoined with a series of arm stretches and body bends that instantly ignites our internal Ki energy. Much refreshed, we are now prepared for the rigorous self-defense and sparring drills that lay ahead. With the assistance of Master Sang Bum Yoon, Jang Ki Park demonstrates a number of effective ho sin sool tactics, intended to disarm, disable, or subdue an attacker. I am grateful to see that the traditional aspects of taekwondo, those of a purely defensive nature, are not dismissed by the attending masters in favor of the sportive elements so prevalent in the martial arts today.

In preparation for WTF-style, full-contact sparring, a training feature favored by many in our group, Master Park's senior, Professor Kyu Seok Lee with one of his most able students in tow, demonstrates the "twenty-five second drill." In this exercise student A, who is the holder, rotates a kicking paddle through the four compass points causing student B, the defender, to circulate within each quadrant while executing a combination of kicking techniques. Anyone attempting this drill for the first time, as well as realizing the value of aerobic conditioning, quickly comes to appreciate the dual roles agility and focus play in taekwondo.

At this point, those wishing to are directed to don fighting gear. Admittedly, it is one thing to spar with students from your own school and another altogether to go eye to eye with some of the world's most elite martial artists. Nevertheless, this is precisely why many of our students elected to visit Korea in the first place: to develop courage in the face of danger while cultivating martial arts skill in harmony with others. Still, how would it go?

Training in Korea: Sparring with the Kyung Won Taekwondo Team

Traveling to Korea, the practitioner can learn valuable lessons from first, second, and now, third-generation native taekwondo masters when the eyes are open and the mind is clear.

We trained at Kyung Won University for several hours, appreciating the gracious hospitality of our hosts. Three members of our group who are eager to take advantage of a unique opportunity to spar elite fighters suit up in full fighting gear, putting on hogu, helmet, arm guards, and shin/instep protectors. A member of our group is facing a wiry student from the Kyung Won Taekwondo Team, perhaps half his age. Both are called to attention by Master Jang Ki Park, our instructor and a professor of taekwondology at the university. Bows of respect are exchanged. Master Park shouts "kyorugi choombi," and both men assume the upright fighting stance. Pulling his hand swiftly back in a front stance, Master Park yells: "sijak!" One thing immediately becomes evident: the Korean martial artists are blindingly fast. This is perhaps the first impression you receive when the sparring begins. Multiple jumping, turning, and thrusting strikes are delivered within fractions of a second. The next obvious thing you cannot help but notice are the kihops that punctuate each technique. These spirit yells not only draw and project Ki from the tanjun, our reservoir of internal energy located two inches below the navel, but in a more practical sense, startle the opponent, causing fear and hesitation to blossom in the heart, while short circuiting concentration.[51]

This speed coupled with the sonic interruption of focus, is a certain recipe for victory both in self-defense and sport sparring. Meanwhile, another one of our students seems to be doing well. He competes regularly in the United States and is a cool competitor. He counters round kicks with jump-turning back kicks and successfully attacks with his premiere technique, the front leg crescent. Time is called. Both fighters bow and embrace one another, proud to have participated in competition of this intensity and quality. The next two matches are fought with equal vigor and all are pleased with the results. However, it is clear that while no overt mention has been made of it, the Koreans appear to be holding back. In truth, this is understandable, in no small part due to the age disparity within the group and a training regimen that requires them to work out continuously each day resulting in unprecedented endurance. Yet, it is evident that the Korean instructors and students realize we are here to learn from them and not merely to compete. As always, taekwondo, regardless of cultural background, is founded on mutual respect.

Again, we are moving via luxury motor coach, our second home-away-from-home, to the Hotel TEMF where we briefly rest and change for the evening. After a full day of hard taekwondo training, we are ready to enjoy the nightlife of Seoul, Korea's capital city with a population of nearly eleven million people. Dinner reservations await us at an officer's club on a local army base. High ranking U.S. and Korean soldiers dressed in crisp uniforms adorned with medals and braids smile and wave when they discover we are American martial artists studying abroad. The festive ambiance is amplified all the more by steins of O.B., a popular Korean beer, that are graciously offered to us by white-jacketed waiters. The restaurant has a decidedly Western flavor and so we choose meat cutlet, a deep-fried breaded steak, from the menu.

Following this delightful meal, we travel a short distance to the Namdaemun Market, a vast open-air maze of alleyways

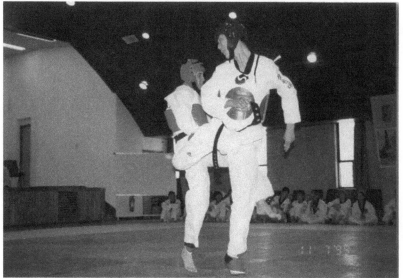

Photo by John Jordan III

Sparring at Kyung Won University.

populated by street vendors and small shops that sell everything from native celadon vases to dried squid, potent ginseng root to fine Asian silk. Haggling is expected and many in our group walk away with unbelievable bargains. Later, we stroll a section of the It'aewon, a strip of hotels, nightclubs, and outlet stores featuring designer clothing, souvenirs, and porcelain goods. I climb a narrow flight of steps to the door of a cramped tailor shop I recall from my last few visits. There, I purchase a black satin jacket and have "Chosun Taekwondo Academy" embroidered on the back while I wait, all for 23,000 *won*, or roughly twenty dollars. By this time I am eager to return to my traditional ondol hotel room where I stretch out on my sleeping mat for a much-needed night's rest.

Six A.M. arrives quickly. My roommate and I jump into our doboks and rush downstairs to the hotel courtyard where Master Sang Bum Yoon is waiting to begin "morning exercises." These informal sessions provide some of the most enjoyable and effective training we will receive during our stay. This is why we chose

151

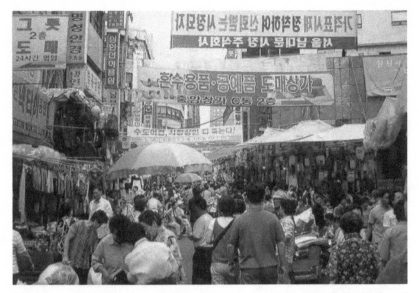

A visit to Namdaemun Market where, within its labyrinth of streets and alleys, anything is available from Koryo celadon to dried squid.

to visit the "Land of the Morning Calm" in the first place, and I am ecstatic!

Exhausted even before the day begins, we return to our rooms where we quickly shower, dress, and prepare for breakfast. Our itinerary calls for an afternoon visit to the Kukkiwon, center of taekwondo operations worldwide. Grandmaster Chun and I, along with two other senior students, are scheduled to meet privately with Dr. Un Yong Kim, the then-president of the Kukkiwon and the WTF. This is an honor beyond imagination, and I am keen on making a positive first impression, especially in the presence of my mentor, Grandmaster Richard Chun.

Training in Korea: The Kukkiwon, World Taekwondo Headquarters

For months we had been anticipating our training and cultural tour of Korea with an intense itinerary calling for a visit to the

Kukkiwon. Located atop a hillside in the Kangnam District of Seoul, the Kukkiwon is home to the World Taekwondo Headquarters. The building itself, reflecting traditional Korean architecture, was constructed in 1972 to house taekwondo-related organizations and to provide taekwondo practitioners with modern training facilities. Besides serving as a center for taekwondo training and competitions, the Kukkiwon, or "National Gymnasium," conducts black belt promotion tests and issues certifications to members of national associations sanctioned by the WTF. The Memorial Museum, established in 1991, positioned the Kukkiwon as the hub of taekwondo culture by depicting the history of the national Korean martial art through related materials. The main training area, management offices, locker rooms, restaurant, gift shop, pavilion for ceremonies, and seminar facilities are all significant components of this sprawling complex.

Upon entering the Kukkiwon, walking amid the hustle and bustle of the crowded hallways, we realize that there is a tournament in progress. Out on the main training floor, black belt students from various educational institutions appear to be competing for a major championship. Just as in any sporting arena,

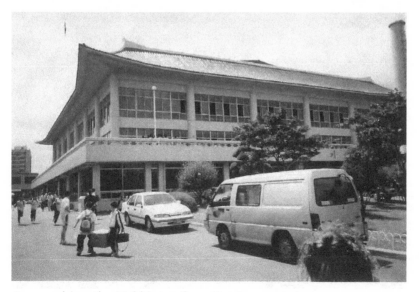

Approaching the Kukkiwon from its steep entryway.

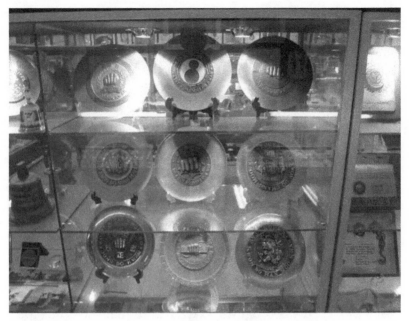

The Kukkiwon Museum where relics, such as these brass plates memorializing the various kwans that were combined to form taekwondo, can be found.

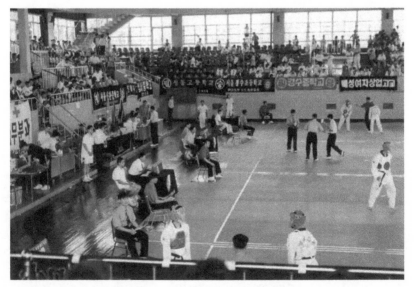

Korean martial artists competing at the Kukkiwon.

the competition area is surrounded by rows of ascending seats. Above the last row, enormous flags are suspended representing the colors of the WTF, the KTA, and of course, the Republic of Korea. The stands are filled with cheering teens and young adults. Our students search for vacant seats so that they may observe the action firsthand. Meanwhile, Grandmaster Chun beckons me to join him and two other senior students who are hurrying down a small staircase. We find ourselves being led through a series of serpentine corridors by an official-looking gentleman in a blue business suit. Suddenly, we are standing before a room accessible only by a set of double wooden doors etched with gold letters announcing the name and office of its occupant: Dr. Un Yong Kim, President, World Taekwondo Federation. The doors open and we are requested to wait in a small anteroom crowded with desks and assorted office equipment. Aides are speaking in hushed tones. Suddenly, an interior door opens and an assistant escorts us into a meeting I can hardly believe is happening.

Even during the early stages of my training, respectful instructors emphasized the importance of being familiar with the organizational structure and hierarchy of taekwondo. All of us as taekwondo practitioners, in some form or another, are related by heritage either through an affiliation with a parent organization, such as the WTF or ITF, or, at minimum, by an undiluted, pure-form practice of taekwondo transmitted by competent master instructors with some connection to Korea. Furthermore, Confucianism, clearly a philosophical paradigm that permeates the Asian martial arts, dictates recognition of seniority. Consequently, the significance of the meeting that is about to occur resonates with these thoughts.

Not long ago, the name of Dr. Un Yong Kim conjured up questions regarding political integrity and sound judgment. Thankfully, this has changed. Dr. Kim is largely responsible for catapulting taekwondo into the international arena using his association with the IOC, coupled with the KTA, as a vehicle. From the creation of the art to the present, he helped clear the way for a provincial system of defensive styles to blossom into the most popular martial art in the world today. To me, he is a giant and I am about to shake his hand through the good offices of my grandmaster.

Dr. Kim's workplace is large by any standard. In the middle, stretches a long, low table surrounded by comfortable, brown leather chairs with cushions sunken with use. Behind is a desk flanked on either side by flags and a cabinet containing mementos from a lifetime of dedicated service to his country, taekwondo, and the IOC. Un Yong Kim's voice is rich and deep, aged by years of negotiations; he is someone who is clearly at home in the halls of power. Immaculately dressed in what appears to be a tailor-made suit, he scrutinizes each of us with eyes that have seen many martial artists. Following a bow and a handshake, he offers us seats and chats freely, welcoming his junior, Richard Chun, to the "Land of the Morning Calm." An assistant enters and hands each of us a large white envelope bearing the stamp of the WTF and the Kukkiwon. We stand and pose for a photograph which, years later, hangs proudly in the entryway of my dojang. Before I realize it, we are ushered, along with Dr. Kim, to an adjoining

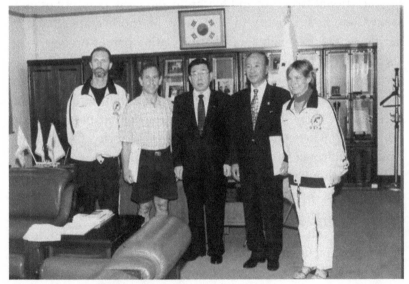

Courtesy of Korea Kukkiwon

An honored meeting with Dr. Un Yong Kim (center) at the Kukkiwon.

seminar room where the remainder of our group awaits, seated at tables and chairs reminiscent of those we are accustomed to seeing in the classroom of an elementary school. Following a brief speech at the microphone, Dr. Kim praises our members for making such a long journey and then passes the podium to Byung Woon Kim, Chairman of the Kukkiwon Technical Subcommittee, who lectures on the history of Olympic-style taekwondo. Later, we pause for yet another photograph, this time with our entire group positioned beneath the ornate hangul lettering that announces the main entrance to the Kukkiwon.

On the bus ride back to the Hotel TEMF, I am eager to discover what is inside my white envelope. I break the seal and am delighted to find a set of cuff links, tie clasp, and wrist watch, all imprinted with the emblem of the WTF—a worthy gift, indeed, from a distinguished man.

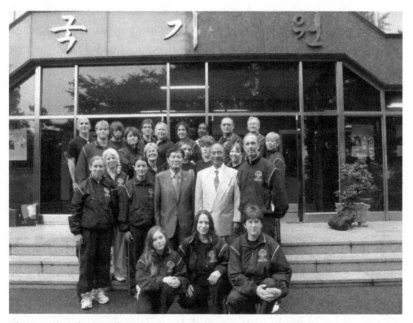

Chosun Taekwondo Academy students pose before the entrance of the Kukkiwon with Grandmaster Richard Chun (center right) and Kukkiwon General Manager Beong Sung Kim (center left) during the 2007 Korea Training & Cultural Tour.

This is my second visit to the Kukkiwon, but my first to enjoy an audience with Dr. Kim. Our journey, thus far, has been a truly enriching experience, and still, it is not ended.

Training in Korea: Visiting the Capital of the Ancient Silla Kingdom

Today our motor coach carries us south to Kyongju, the ancient capital of the Silla Kingdom and the training ground of the Hwarang, Korea's ancient warrior-elite that devoted much time to the practice of the martial arts underscored by an appreciation for Asian philosophy and ethical behavior in battle.

We rumble along the four hundred fifty kilometer Gyeong-Bu Expressway, the first built in modern Korea, connecting Seoul to Busan. Traveling at a constant eighty miles per hour, the trip will take roughly five hours. I cannot help but recall the emotions, I, a foreigner, experienced one sunny summer morning years ago while driving south along this very roadway. As I gazed out the tinted glass window of our motor coach, the picturesque scenery could not erase the thought that a few short decades ago the serenity of this place had been shattered by the atrocities of war. Whether the invading Communist forces had actually taken this route in pushing the South Koreans back to the apparent safety of the Busan perimeter was irrelevant at the time. For in doing the research for my last two books I knew only too well that the entire country had been indiscriminately soaked with blood in a war between brothers and sisters of the same parent nation. More disturbing, however, was the thought that this onerous division remains to this day with only a whisper of resolution in sight.

Fortunately, the leisurely ride allows me time to sit and speak at length with Grandmaster Chun concerning the philosophy of taekwondo and his unique outlook on teaching mature students. He reminds me that *purpose in practice* is of the utmost importance coupled with the precise performance of poomsae.[52] Following our invaluable discussion, I moved to the front of the bus with Nikon camera in hand. I snap a photo of a particularly interesting tunnel featuring a depiction of two characters with flowing hair carefully etched on its entrance. Its seems everything along this road has a mystical character all its own, from the traditional tile-roofed houses nestled beside terraced rice fields to the small ancestral cemeteries and shrines dotting the countryside.

Before we know it, our motor coach lazily negotiates a banked exit ramp and proceeds through an ornate toll plaza complete with a sign announcing in large letters that we have arrived in Kyongju. Our first stop is Tumuli Park, where great mounds of earth mark the tombs of ancient Silla royalty. It was here in 1974 that Chon'mach'ong, the Flying Horse Tomb, was excavated yielding more than ten thousand treasures including a golden crown adorned with kidney-shaped jade, traditionally worn by the Sillian kings. Upon the monarch's death, he, along with many of his worldly possessions, was placed in a room-like enclosure. Gravel, rock, and then earth were piled on top eventually creating the fifty foot, semi-spherical shapes before us. This ingenious method of construction discouraged looting since the

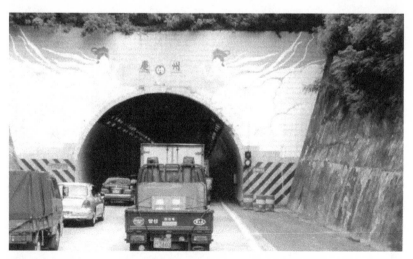

Paintings of enchanting characters grace the entrance of a tunnel on the Gyeong-Bu Expressway.

only safe entry was from the top of the mound thus eliminating surreptitious entry from below.

A short distance from the tombs, we find Ch'omsongdae Observatory. Built during the seventh century, this bottle-shaped building is thought to be the oldest structure of its kind in the world. Legend has it that Sillian queens would be lifted through the small, south-facing rectangular opening to gaze at the heavens. From here we move to the luxurious, five-star Concord Hotel where we relax and dine before turning in for the evening. My roommate, John Jordan III and I have again chosen a traditional ondol room and the hard floor beneath the sleeping mat feels good on my back.

Next morning, following our sunrise training with Master Sang Bum Yoon and a deluxe, Western-style breakfast of eggs, bacon, and strong coffee, we venture to Bulguksa Temple. Originally built in A.D. 353, it is a stunning monument to both the skill of Silla's architects and its Buddhist faith. We are humbled by the splendor of the tiled roofs supported by timeless timbers painted

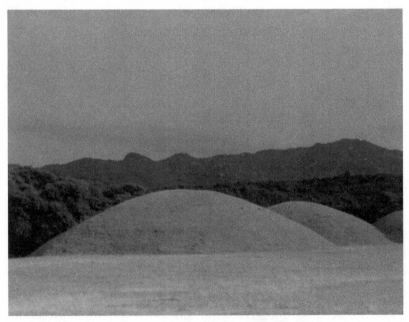

Tumuli Park, final resting place of Sillian royalty.

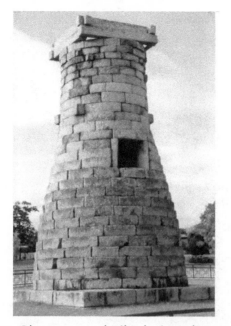

Ch'omsongdae Observatory, built during the seventh century, where from the square opening, Sillian queens would gaze at the heavens.

in the brilliant blue, green, and red hues unique to temple art. Our students seize the moment since this is the perfect setting for a series of dignified photos depicting the beauty and strength of traditional taekwondo. Grandmaster Chun and I pose together in the horse stance with a temple entrance as a backdrop, he, executing a double mountain block and I, a double spread block. Later, to our delight, we discover that the monks in permanent residence have given us permission to join them for a period of meditation. Removing our shoes, we bow and enter the relative dark of an ancient meditation hall. The surrounding air hangs heavy with a sense of peace mixed with the twisting wisps of sandalwood incense. A great gold statue of the Buddha sits before us and time disappears as we attempt to relinquish all thought . . . at least for now.

Before we know it, our trip has ended and we are on our way to Kimpo International Airport. Images of the past week play across our mind like a slideshow. Aside from the incredible technical knowledge we have gained, friends have been made and enduring memories created that will last a lifetime. Clearly, by visiting the elegant temples, shrines, and academic institutions

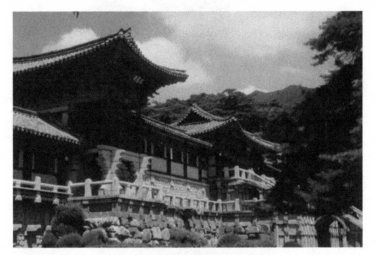

Bulguksa Temple, a stunning example of Sillian architecture.

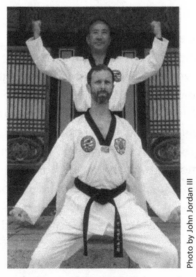

Grandmaster Richard Chun (top) with his senior student Master Doug Cook at Bulguksa Temple in Kyongju, South Korea.

dedicated to the birth and development of the native martial arts, we not only begin to feel a physical connection to taekwondo, but a geographical and chronological attraction as well. It is my sincere belief that any practitioner wishing to embrace taekwondo in its fullness needs to plan a pilgrimage to Korea: "Land of the Morning Calm."

What Do We Do Now?

I have just returned from leading the most recent Chosun Taekwondo Academy Training & Cultural Tour of Korea along with Grandmaster Richard Chun and, barring the jetlag, found our experiences in the homeland of taekwondo almost beyond words. Indeed, each time I revisit Korea, I see deeper into the traditions and customs that influenced the creation of the world's most popular martial art. During this excursion, our instruction ran the gamut from kicking drills at Yong-In University outside of Seoul to a monastic meal and intense training in *sunmudo* with Buddhist monk/martial artists at Golgusa Temple high in the clouds atop the mountains surrounding the Kyongju plain. Yet, since many in our group appreciate poomsae and realize the important role they play in delineating traditional taekwondo as the classical martial art that it is, the time spent in the tiny village of Yangsu-ri with Grandmaster Gyoo Hyun Lee at his dojang surrounded by rice paddies will likely remain the most memorable. It warmed my heart to see Grandmaster Chun and Grandmaster Lee—both world-renowned 9th dan black belts—meet for the first time.

After I entered Grandmaster Lee's newly-built dojang with breathtaking views of the valley below, I quickly changed into my dobok. Taking my place in line, we assumed the *joombi* stance, bowed, and the training session officially began. The nervous anticipation our group was projecting immediately shattered as a smiling, middle-aged master instructor who was assisting Grandmaster Lee began the standard warm up and flexibility exercises. Many of the more extreme postures were borrowed from

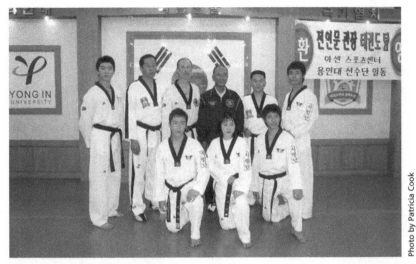

Photo by Patricia Cook

Members of the Yong-In University Taekwondo Team with Grand-master Richard Chun (center right) and the author (center left).

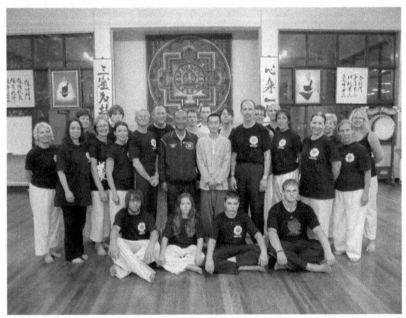

Photo by Patricia Cook

Participants during the 2007 Chosun Taekwondo Academy Korea Training & Cultural Tour practiced traditional Korean Zen martial arts at Golgusa Temple overlooking the vast Kyongju Plain.

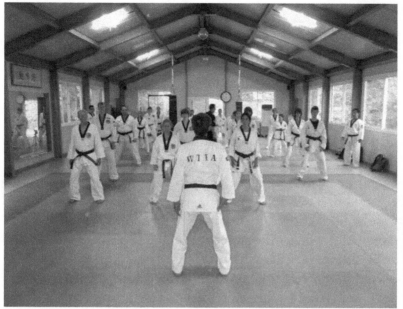

Photo by Patricia Cook

Grandmaster Gyoo Hyun Lee prepares Chosun Taekwondo Academy students for an intense training session focusing on poomsae.

hatha yoga and we began to perspire as the heat from our bodies warmed the room. We continued working on technique that many would accuse of being far too simple in exchange for an eight-thousand mile trip. Yet my students and I were so intrigued when the grandmaster reviewed the process of making a proper fist that we photographed the precision with which it was accomplished along with the wear and tear on the fist that is a result of striking solid objects for many years. Basic technique followed with our front stance, back stance, middle blocks, knife hand blocks, front kicks, round and side kicks, scrutinized beneath the magnifying glass of experience. A common thread running through the execution of every strike or block was the constant reminder to relax in our delivery and tense at the point of impact or penetration of the target.

After several hours of uninterrupted training, a break was called and we congregated in small groups to compare notes and review what we were taught. The conversation turned to differences some were noticing in the fabric of instruction. However, before I could gain a better understanding of the root of these questions, we were commanded to reconvene.

Following the obligatory bows of respect, we were separated into groups according to belt rank and prepared for poomsae practice. Thinking back, in comparison to prior visits, I could not have been more delighted with the direction our training had taken over the course of the last few days of our trip. In candid discussions with several Korean practitioners during my visits, I was told of a movement by a number of master instructors who were initiating a return from a strictly sportive approach to a more holistic style of training, including forms and self-defense drills. Our experiences that day, and the days previous, seemed to confirm the reality of this trend. Although the Palgwe set was not given credence, the eight Taegeuk forms, in tandem with the mandatory WTF black belt series poomsae, were thankfully addressed in great detail. For the black belts and color belts alike, no banquet was as bountiful as that day's forms practice; each of us was afforded the opportunity to refine the basic skills contained within the poomsae unique to belt level, either under the intense direction of Grandmaster Lee or one of his accomplished instructors. I was working on poomsae Sipjin while other black belts were focusing on Keumgang and Koryo. Patiently, Grandmaster Lee explained the practical application of each movement of my form in conjunction with its proper trajectory and chamber. Meanwhile, from the corner of my eye, I glimpsed my students receiving equal attention in analyzing the various Taegeuk poomsae, albeit with some minor alterations from what they were accustomed to.

As the day progressed, a potential dilemma began to gnaw at me as it must many instructors from time to time, and I sensed what it was my students were referring to earlier as "differences" in curriculum. The World Taekwondo Instructor Academy, under the direction of Grandmaster Gyoo Hyun Lee, is attempting, at least on the surface, to introduce a subtle shift in the dynamic

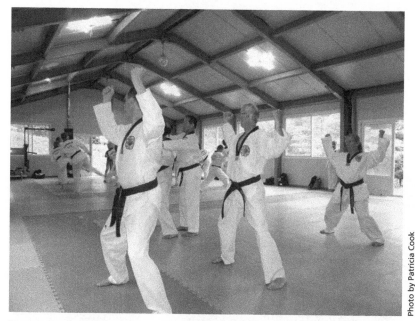

Photo by Patricia Cook

Doug Cook (left) James Vandenburg Jr. (center), Cheryl Crouchen (rear), and Erica Linthorst (right) practice Keumgang under the stern eye of Grandmaster Gyoo Hyun Lee at his dojang in Yangsu-ri, South Korea.

principles of taekwondo technique based on an advanced understanding of physics as it relates to body mechanics. A modern approach, authored by Grandmaster Lee and other native Korean masters, is being applied to footwork, power ratio, chambering, and weapons training, while at the same time, attempting to maintain the value of traditionalism. On that rainy afternoon in the tiny village of Yangsu-ri, we were exposed to technical variations that faintly contradicted the manner of execution we are familiar with, forcing my students to politely ask: "What do we do now?"

Buried in this question is an important lesson both for me and my colleagues. Traditional taekwondo is a cultural treasure chest filled with effective self-defense skills supported by a virtuous philosophy. Although the Korean discipline contains immutable tools such as the round kick, back fist, and knife hand block, to name a few, the manner in which these are performed may vary slightly from master to master. This fact does not corrupt the basic principles of taekwondo; rather, it adds color and individuality to something that is an art rather than an absolute science. Consequently, it is my desire to expose my students, at least those capable of sustaining an open mind, to the diversity inherent in taekwondo, resulting in what I hope will be perceived as an enhanced training experience overall. Having said this, however, it is to the teachings of my instructor, Grandmaster Richard Chun, that I am faithful. Time and time again he has proven to be a loyal proponent of the technical heritage of taekwondo, while remaining respectful of progress. In that tradition, I wish to provide my students with an expanded worldview of our practice while simultaneously remaining steadfast to the values and technical elements that I have been gifted with over the decades. So in answer to the question: "What do we do now?"—we continue on as we have been taught, adding and retaining what our seniors feel is valuable while remaining respectful of the differences others apply. This is the tradition of what we do. It is the manner in which we learn. It is *The Way* of taekwondo . . . a path to excellence.

Last Words

Taekwondo is an Ocean with No Horizon . . .
Continue the Journey

Glossary

Aikido	The Way of Harmonizing Ki, a Japanese martial art relying on a system of throws and locks in conjunction with the redirection of an opponent's negative energy
Akum sohn	Arc hand, alligator hand, or tiger mouth technique
Baljitki	Footwork
Beginner's Mind	A Zen Buddhist concept, an innocent and open outlook on practice and life in general
Bom sogi	Cat or tiger stance
Bong	Wooden fighting staff
Chang-Han	"Blue Cottage," a set of twenty four tul of patterns unique to the International Tae-kwon-Do Federation
Cha Riot	Attention stance
Chon-Ji	The first of twenty four tul in the Chang-Han set, unique to the International Tae-kwon-Do Federation
Dan	Black belt degree level
Dobok	The V-neck style uniform worn exclusively by the taekwondoist.
Dojang	A place to study *The Way*; a training hall unique to the Korean martial arts
Dwiro dora	About face
Ee Su Sik	Two-step sparring
Gi	The traditional wrap-around uniform used primarily in the Japanese martial arts

Ge-Baek	The twelfth of twenty four tul or patterns unique to the International Taekwon-Do Federation; also a famous general of the Paekche Kingdom
Gungfu	Literally, "hard work" or "good effort," a generic term for the Chinese martial arts. (Also spelled kung-fu)
Gup	Color belt grade level.
Hanbok	A type of traditional Korean clothing
Hwarang	An elite group of young warriors that lived during the Silla dynasty
Hwarang-do	"Way of the Flowering Manhood"
Hogu	Chest protector used in sparring
Ho Sin Sool	Self-defense or self-protection method
I Ching	The ancient Taoist *Book of Changes* used as an oracle for centuries by those seeking metaphysical guidance
Il Su Sik	One-step sparring
Hatha Yoga	An Eastern discipline that utilizes physical exercises and breath work to achieve flexibility and spiritual enrichment coupled with a sense of well being
Hongik-ingan	Korean philosophy supporting the benefits of universal humanism
Hyung	Category. A traditional term for a series of choreographed defensive and offensive techniques aimed at defeating multiple attackers coming from different directions. (See Poomsae, Tul, and Kata)
Ilyo	Last in a series of nine black belt poomsae unique to the World Taekwondo Federation and the Kukkiwon

Ja choom sogi	Horse stance
Jaese-ikwa	Korean philosophy advocating the rationalization of human living
Jeet Kune Do	"The Way of the Intercepting Fist," a martial art developed by the late Bruce Lee
Jingol	Sillian citizen of true-bone status
Joombi	Ready stance
Judo	"The Gentle Way," a Japanese martial art and Olympic sport centering on throws and sweeps developed by Jigoro Kano in 1882
Judoka	A judo practitioner
Kata	A Japanese term to describe a series of choreographed defensive and offensive techniques aimed at defeating multiple attackers coming from different directions (See Poomsae, Hyung, and Tul)
Kang Sang Koon	A traditional Korean black belt poomsae, also known as Kum Sang Gang
Keumgang	Second in a series of nine black belt poomsae unique to the World Taekwondo Federation and the Kukkiwon
Ki	The universal life force used by the martial artist to amplify technique
Kibon	Basics; also a set of five traditional poomsae
Kicho	A set of three basic forms designated for beginners
Kihon	Japanese term for basics
Kihop	Spirit yell; the verbal projection of Ki used by the martial artist to amplify technique

Kong Soo Do	"Empty-Hand-Way," an early name given to one of the indigenous hard-style Korean martial arts that eventually developed in taekwondo
Koryo	First in a series of nine black belt poomsae unique to the World Taekwondo Federation and the Kukkiwon; a dynasty existing on the Korean peninsula from A.D. 918 to 1392
Koryo celadon	A type of ceramic bearing a unique green, blue, or white glaze developed by artisans during the Koryo dynasty
Kukson	National seniors or officers of the Hwarang
Kumite	Japanese term for sparring
Kyuk Pa	The breaking of solid objects to promote penetrating power and focus.
Kwonbop	Fist-Fighting Method
Kyorugi	Sparring
Kyorugi joombi	Sparring ready stance
Kyungye	The bow of respect
Machueo kyorugi	Prearranged sparring
Momtong jiluki	Middle punch
Moo Duk Kwan	The Institute of Martial Virtue founded in 1945 by Hwang Kee
Mudra	Sanskrit term meaning "to seal in," a hand gesture used in meditation
Mushin	A Japanese term for "empty mind"
Ondol	A traditional Korean room usually with a heated floor

Poomsae	Movements of motions. A series of choreographed defensive and offensive techniques aimed at defeating multiple attackers coming from different directions. (See Tul, Hyung, and Kata)
Pyongwon	Fourth in a series of nine black belt poomsae unique to the World Taekwondo Federation and the Kukkiwon
Pyung-Ahn	A set of five traditional patterns derived from the Pinan set meaning balance and confidence
Qigong	An ancient Chinese healing art based on the manipulation and balancing of Qi or Ki
Sabumnim	Master black belt, 4th dan or above
Sam Su Sik	Three-step sparring
Samgeuk	A yellow, blue, and red spiral symbolizing humanity, earth, and heaven
Samsilshingo	Philosophical concept describing the foundation of the universe composed of heaven, earth and humanity
Sensei	Japanese term for teacher
Seon	Philosophical concept of impeccable goodness or virtue; also defined as Zen
Seonggol	Sillian king or queen of sacred bone status
Sifu	Chinese term for teacher
Sijak	Begin
Sipjin	Fifth in a series of nine black belt poomsae unique to the World Taekwondo Federation and the Kukkiwon
Subyeokta	An ancient martial discipline using the hands, arms, and legs as swords

Taebaek	Third in a series of nine black belt poomsae unique to the World Taekwondo Federation and the Kukkiwon
Taegeuk Chil Jang	Seventh in a series of eight color belt poomsae unique to the World Taekwondo federation and the Kukkiwon
Taegeuk Sa Jang	Fourth in a series of eight color belt poomsae unique to the World Taekwondo federation and the Kukkiwon
Taegeuk Yook Jang	Sixth in a series of eight color belt poomsae unique to the World Taekwondo federation and the Kukkiwon
Taekwondo	"Foot-Hand-Way," the traditional martial art and Olympic sport of Korea
Taesoodo	"Kick-Fist-Way," an early term given to the Korean martial art that would eventually evolve into *taekwondo*
Taijichuan	"Grand Ultimate Fist," an internal Chinese martial art influenced by the principles of the *I Ching*, practiced primarily to promote health and well being
Tangoon	The mythical progenitor of Korea thought to have lived in 2333 B.C.
Tangsoodo	"The Way of the China Hand," a traditional Korean martial art predating *taekwondo* but active today
Tanjun	The body's Ki or energy center located two inches below the navel
Tong-Il	The last of twenty four tul or patterns unique to the International Taekwon-Do Federation

Tul	Patterns. A traditional term to describe a series of choreographed defensive and offensive techniques aimed at defeating multiple attackers coming from different directions. (See Poomsae, Hyung, and Kata)
Wushu	Modern Chinese competition martial art derived from kungfu
Yudanja	Referring to dan grade or black belt as in the case of the nine WTF black belt poomsae

Notes

1. *Taekwondo as an Instrument for Peace,* Chungwon Choue. www.peace-sports.org
2. There are more than 3,000 fundamental movements in Taekwon-Do, and General Choi was very proud of this. These movements are basic elements that can be likened to musical notes; when linked, they produce a harmonious result. www.tkd-itf.org; *Original Taekwon-Do e-Magazine* 2 (August 2009): 15, found at www.tkd-itf.co.uk
3. *Promise and Fulfillment in the Art of Taekwondo.* Sang Kyu Shim. Self-Published, 1974, p. 20.
4. Internet Reference—www.wikipedia.org—Just more than 40 percent of South Koreans profess religious affiliation. That affiliation is spread among a great variety of traditions, including Buddhism (34 percent), Christianity (30 percent), Confucianism (0.2 percent), and Shamanism.
5. *A New History of Korea,* Ki Baik Lee. Harvard University Press, 1984, pp. 380-81.
6. *Korea's Place in the Sun,* Bruce Cummings. Norton & Co., 1997, pp. 303-4.
7. "People & Events in Taekwondo's Formative Years," Dakin Burdick. *Journal of Asian Martial Arts,* Vol. 6 #1, 1997, p. 41.
8. For a comprehensive history regarding the formative years of taekwondo see *Traditional Taekwondo: Core Techniques, History and Philosophy,* Doug Cook. YMAA Publication Center, 2006, pp. 19-29.
9. *The I Ching* or *Book of Changes,* translated by Hellmut Wilhelm with a foreword by C. G. Jung. Princeton University Press, 1967. One of the more frequently recommended versions of this book.
10. *Advancing in Taekwondo,* Richard Chun. YMAA Publication Center, 2006, pp. 136-358.
11. For an in-depth explanation of *hapkido* see *Hapkido: Traditions, Philosophy, Technique,* Marc Tedeschi. Weatherhill, 2000.
12. Philosophy of the dobok is described by the Korea Taekwondo Association: www.koreataekwondo.org
13. *Taekwondo—Philosophy & Culture,* Kyong Myong Lee. Hollym, 2001, p. 42.
14. *Kukkiwon Textbook.* O Sung Publishing Company, 2006, p. 636.
15. *Advancing in Tae Kwon Do,* Richard Chun. YMAA Publication Center, 2006, p. 28.
16. *Ki: A Practical Guide for Westerners.* William Reed. Japan Publications, 1986, p. 19.
17. *The Making of the Martial Artist,* Sang Kyu Shim. TKD Enterprises, 1980. Foreword.
18. Mark Salzman's *Iron and Silk,* published by Vintage, is a delightful and entertaining read describing his adventures while training and teaching in China.
19. *Korea the Beautiful: Treasures of the Hermit Kingdom,* Yushin Yoo. Golden Pond Press, 1987, p. 82.
20. Kukkiwon Textbook. O Sung Publishing Company, 2006, p. 58.
21. Internet Reference—www.wikipedia.org—The *Samguk Yusa,* or *Memorabilia of the Three Kingdoms,* is a collection of legends, folktales, and

historical accounts relating to the Three Kingdoms of Korea, as well as to other periods and states before, during, and after the Three Kingdoms period.

22. *The History of Taekwondo Patterns*, Richard Mitchell. Lilley Gulch, 1987, p. 63.

23. Another legend I am aware of, but the source is unknown to me.

24. *Politics: Who Gets What When How*, Harold Dwight Lasswell. Meridian. 1958.

25. "General Choi Hong Hi: A Taekwon-Do History Lesson," *Tae Kwon Do Times*. He Young Kim, January, 2000, Vol. 20 #1, p. 46.

26. *Tae Kwon Do: The Ultimate Reference Guide to the World's Most Popular Martial Art*, Yeon Hee Park, Hwan Yeon Park, and Jon Gerrard. Checkmark Books, 1989.

27. The *Analects of Confucius* profess a reciprocal relationship between the individual, family, community, and state.

28. *Taekwondo – Philosophy & Culture*, Kyong Myong Lee. Hollym, 2001, p. 22.

29. "People & Events in Taekwondo's Formative Years," Dakin Burdick. *Journal of Asian Martial Arts*, Vol. 6 #1, 1997.

30. *Traditional Taekwondo—Core Techniques, History, and Philosophy*, Doug Cook. YMAA Publication Center, 2006, p. 84.

31. "General Choi Hong Hi: A Taekwon-Do History Lesson," *Tae Kwon Do Times*. He Young Kim. January, 2000, Vol. 20 #1, p. 50.

32. The *kihop* or spirit yell, is used by the martial artist to amplify technique and channel Ki energy.

33. Marc Tedeschi's book *Essential Anatomy*, Weatherhill, 2000, charts in detail the various vital points and meridians to target on the human body.

34. This event occurred at Kyung Won University in 1999 during a training tour of Korea. Grandmaster Kyu Seok Lee felt one of his students was under-achieving and disciplined him in this manner.

35. Haddock Taekwondo is located in the Sokol School at 420 East 71 Street in New York City.

36. Promotion test periods vary from school to school. Most schools hold examinations every quarter while some test every two months; black belt dan test periods range in years.

37. Specials have appeared on public television depicting Shaolin monks resisting harm through the use of Ki from a metal rod pressed against the throat.

38. Both *il su sik* and *ho sin sool* techniques should be practiced from the left and right sides to prove effective in any situation.

39. For a list of the current essay assignments required by our school, visit the Chosun Taekwondo Academy website at: www.chosuntkd.com

40. To this day I still retain my color belt essays along with sweat-stained notes I used to learn new poomsae.

41. The Chosun Taekwondo Academy is an affiliate school of the United States Taekwondo Association under the direction of Grandmaster Richard Chun.

42. Internet Reference—www.wikipedia.org—In 2004, the Bruce Lee Foundation decided to use the name *Jun Fan Jeet Kune Do* to refer to the martial arts system that Lee founded. "*Jun Fan*" was Lee's Chinese given name, so the literal translation is "*Bruce Lee's Way of the Intercepting Fist.*"

43. Hwang Kee tells of teaching his style of Korean martial arts in railroad stations where he was employed. Korean masters who immigrated to Tokyo during the

Japanese Occupation of Korea are said to have trained on the rooftop of a local gym.

44. This concept is attributed to one of my senior students, Elizabeth Quasius, who said, "Taekwondo is like a gift to be opened every day."

45. Following his retirement, the Richard Chun Taekwondo Center closed its doors in 2004. Grandmaster Chun, however, continues to travel the country teaching seminars along with his many loyal instructors.

46. *Moving Zen,* C. W. Nicol. Quill, 1975, p. 42.

47. For information regarding group taekwondo tours to Korea, contact the Chosun Taekwondo Academy at www.chosuntkd.com or the Korea Tourism Organization (KTO) at www.visitkorea.or.kr

48. On several occasions during our visits to Korea, my students and I have been known to consume baby octopus, grasshoppers, and silkworm larvae.

49. Once, while training at Kyung Won University, we were directed to run two miles up a steep mountain and back down again following this series of aerobic exercises.

50. *Taekwondo—Ancient Wisdom for the Modern Warrior,* Doug Cook. YMAA Publication Center, 2001, pp. 197-204.

51. The *tanjun,* or Ki center, can be thought of as a small star radiating energy throughout the body. Extracted from the breath, it is the place where Ki is stored.

52. Refer to *The Practice of Purpose in Taekwondo* section in this book.

Bibliography

Burdick, Dakin. "People & Events in Taekwondo's Formative Years," *Journal of Asian Martial Arts* 6, no. 1 (1997): 41.

Chou, Chungwon. *Taekwondo as an Instrument for Peace.* www.peace-sports.org

Chun, Rhin Moon Richard. *Advancing in Taekwondo.* Boston: YMAA, 2007.

———. *Moo Duk Kwan Taekwondo.* California: Ohara Publishing, 1983.

———. *Taekwondo—A Korean Martial Art.* Boston: YMAA, 2007.

———. *Taekwondo—Spirit and Practice.* Boston: YMAA, 2003.

Cook, Doug. *Taekwondo—Ancient Wisdom for the Modern Warrior.* Boston: YMAA, 2001.

———. *Traditional Taekwondo—Core Techniques, History, and Philosophy.* Boston: YMAA, 2006.

Cummings, Bruce. *Korea's Place in the Sun.* New York: Norton & Co., 1997.

Deshimaru, Taisen. *Zen Way to the Martial Arts.* New York: Penguin Books, 1982.

Funakoshi, Gichin. *Karate-Do Kyohan.* Tokyo: Kodansha Int'l, 1973.

Hyams, Joe. *Zen in the Martial Arts.* New York: Bantam Book, 1979.

I Ching or *Book of Changes,* translated by Hellmut Wilhelm with a foreword by Carl G. Jung. New Jersey: Princeton UP, 1967.

International Taekwon-do Federation. "General Choi, Hong Hi: Founder of Taekwondo." www.tkd-itf.org

Kauz, Herman. *The Martial Spirit.* New York: Overlook Press, 1977.

Kee, Hwang. *Tang Soo Do.* New Jersey: Sang Moon Sa, 1978.

Kukkiwon. *Kukkiwon Textbook.* Seoul: Oh-Sung Publishing, 2006.

Kim, Daeshik. *One-Step Sparring.* Seoul: NANAM Publishing, 1985.

———. *Taekwondo.* Seoul: NANAM Publishing, 1991.

Kim, He Young. "General Choi Hong Hi: A Taekwon-Do History Lesson," *Tae Kwon Do Times* 20, no. 1 (January, 2000): 46, 50.

Kim, Un Yong. *The Taekwon-Do Textbook.* Korea: Oh-Sung Publishing, 1995.

Lasswell, Harold Dwight. *Politics: Who Gets What When How.* New York: Meridian, 1958.

Lee, Ki Baik. *A New History of Korea.* Cambridge: Harvard UP, 1984.

Lee, Kyong Myong. *Taekwondo—Philosophy & Culture.* Seoul and NJ: Hollym, 2001.

LeShan, Lawrence. *How to Meditate.* New York: Bantam Books, 1974.

Losik, Len. *The Kwans of Tang Soo Do.* California: SanLen Publishing, 2003.

Mitchell, Richard L. *The History of Taekwondo Patterns.* Littleton, CO: Lilley Gulch TKD, 1987.

Morgan, Forrest E. *Living the Martial Way.* Ft. Lee, New Jersey: Barricade Books, 1992.

Nicol, C. W. *Moving Zen: One Man's Journey to the Heart of Karate.* California, London, Milan, and Tokyo: Kodansha Int'l: 2001.

Park, Yeon Hee, Yeon Hwan Park, and Jon Gerrard. *Taekwondo: The Ultimate Guide to the World's Most Popular Martial Art.* New York: Facts on File, 1986.

Reed, William. *Ki: A Practical Guide for Westerners.* Tokyo: Japan Publications, 1986.

Salzman, Mark. *Iron and Silk*. New York: Vintage, 1986.

Shim, Sang Kyu. *Promise and Fulfillment in the Art of Taekwondo*. [Self-published] (N.p: n.p.), 1974.

Shim, Sang Kyu and Leo Knight. *The Making of a Martial Artist*. Cedar Rapids, Iowa: TKD Enterprises, 1980.

Suzuki, Shonryu. *Zen Mind, Beginner's Mind*. New York: Weatherhill Inc., 1970.

Tedeschi, Marc. *Essential Anatomy*. Trumble, CT: Weatherhill, Inc., 2001.

———. *Hapkido: Traditions, Philosophy, Technique*. New York: Weatherhill, 2000.

Tokitsu, Kenji. *Ki and the Way of the Martial Arts*. Boston: Shambhala, 2003.

Tohei, Koichi. *Ki in Daily Life*. Tokyo: Japan Publications, 1978.

Wei, Wu. *I-Ching Life: Living it*. California: Power Press, 1996.

Yang, Jwing-Ming. *Qigong for Health and Martial Arts*. Boston: YMAA,1985.

Yoo, Yushin. *Korea the Beautiful: Treasures of the Hermit Kingdom*. Los Angeles and Louisiana: Golden Pond Press, 1987.

Organization, Addresses, and Web Sites

The Kukkiwon: 635, Yoksam-dong, Kangnam-gu, Seoul, Korea 135-908 www.kukkiwon.or.kr

The World Taekwondo Federation: 4F Joyang Building 113, Samseong-dong Gangnam-gu, Seoul, Korea 134-090 www.wtf.org

The United States Taekwondo Association: 87 Stonehurst Drive, Tenafly, NJ 07670 USA www.usta.info

The International Taekwon-Do Federation: Via Cesare Pascoletti 29, scala A2, interno F, 00163 Rome, Italy www.tkd-itf.org

The International Taekwon-do Federation: Yiewsley Leisure Centre, Otterfield Road, Yiewsley, United Kingdom UB7 8 PE www.itf-administration.com/

The International Taekwon-do Federation: Draugasse 3, 1210 Vienna, Austria www.itftkd.org/

The Korea Taekwondo Association: Olympic Park, 88-2 Oryun-dong, Songpa-gu, Seoul, Korea www.koreataekwondo.org

TaeKwonDo Times Magazine: 3950 Wilson Ave SW, Cedar Rapids, IA 52404 USA www.taekwondotimes.com

The Chosun Taekwondo Academy: 62 Main Street, Warwick, NY 10990 USA www.chosuntkd.com

YMAA Publication Center: P.O. Box 480, 23 N. Main St., Suite C, Wolfeboro, NH 03894 USA www.ymaa.com

Index

About the Author

Master Doug Cook holds a 5th dan black belt in the Korean martial art of taekwondo and is certified as an instructor and in rank by the United States Taekwondo Association and the Kukkiwon. After training in Korea on several occasions, he went on to become a six-time gold medalist in the New York State Championships and the New York State Governor's Cup Competitions. He holds a D3 status as a U.S. Referee and has received high honors from Korea in the form of a "Letter of Appreciation" signed 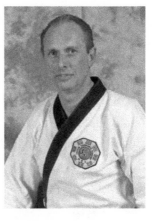 by World Taekwondo Federation president, Dr. Un Yong Kim. In 2003 Doug Cook was awarded the Medal of Special Recognition from the Moo Duk Kwan in Seoul, South Korea. In 2004 while attending a training camp in Korea, he received a Special Citation from the Korean government for forging a stronger relationship between Korea and the United States through the martial arts. A six-page interview appeared in the May 2005 issue of *Tae Kwon Do Times* focusing on taekwondo philosophy and his views on the role the martial arts will play in the twenty-first century. In June 2006, he was inducted into the Budo International Martial Arts Hall of Fame as "Taekwondo Master of the Year." In 2007 he was invited on several occasions to speak as a guest lecturer at the University of Bridgeport in Connecticut, the only institution of higher learning in the country to offer a major in the martial arts. He was recently listed in *Black Belt* magazine as one of the "Top Twenty Masters of the Korean Martial Arts in America." In 2009 he was invited to speak at the prestigious Korea Society in New York City and will appear in *Legacy*, an upcoming television documentary on taekwondo scheduled for release in 2010.

Master Cook and his students are credited with the creation of the Chosun Women's Self-Defense Course. He has also provided training for the U.S. Army National Guard/42d Division prior to military operations and currently instructs agents from the Department of

Homeland Security, the New York Police Department, and the Bronx County Sheriff's Department. He was called upon to demonstrate taekwondo as part of a three-man team at the annual Oriental World of Self-Defense held in New York City's famed Madison Square Garden. There, he and his team were cheered on by martial arts legends Richard Chun, Henry Cho, and Chuck Norris.

Because he is a traditionalist, Master Cook places great emphasis on the underlying philosophical principles and self-defense strategies surrounding taekwondo. He demonstrates this belief by infusing practical meditation, breathing exercises, a strong attention to basics, and the practice of the classical forms, or poomsae, in his instructional methodology.

Aside from continuing his martial arts education under the tutelage of world-renowned, 9th dan black belt Grandmaster Richard Chun, Master Cook owns and operates the Chosun Taekwondo Academy located in Warwick, New York, an institute specializing in traditional martial arts instruction and Ki, or internal energy, development. Master Cook currently shares his knowledge of taekwondo through a series of articles he has written for *TaeKwonDo Times*, *Black Belt* magazine, and the *United States Taekwondo Association Journal*, as well as various other martial arts publications. He also writes a monthly column for *TaeKwonDo Times* entitled "Traditions." In addition to this book, *Taekwondo—A Path to Excellence*, he is the author of two best-selling books focusing on taekwondo entitled, *Taekwondo—Ancient Wisdom for the Modern Warrior* and *Traditional Taekwondo—Core Techniques, History, and Philosophy*, a finalist in *ForeWord* magazine's Book of the Year Award. All editions are published by YMAA Publication Center, Inc., and are available online and at booksellers throughout the world. Master Doug Cook can be reached via email at chosuntkd@yahoo.com and is available for seminars, workshops, and lectures. His web address is www.chosuntkd.com

BOOKS FROM YMAA

DVDS FROM YMAA

more products available from . . .

YMAA Publication Center, Inc. 楊氏東方文化出版中心

1-800-669-8892 • info@ymaa.com • www.ymaa.com

Printed in the USA
CPSIA information can be obtained
at www.ICGtesting.com
JSHW021739060923
47941JS00001B/161

9 781594 391286